SLIMMING TECHNIQUES

SLIMMING TECHNIQUES

PARVESH HANDA

GYAN

GYAN PUBLISHING HOUSE

NEW DELHI-110002

This book is reference only, not as a medical guide or manual of self-treatment. No treatment should be taken without consultation of doctor

Slimming Techniques

Rs. 690

ISBN: 81-212-0912-9

Published in 2006 in India by
Gyan Publishing House
5, Ansari Road, Darya Ganj,
New Delhi-110002
Phones : 23282060, 23261060
Fax : 011-23285914
E-mail : books@ gyanbooks.com
Website: www.gyanbooks.com

Lassertype Setting by: Rudra Computer Graphics, Delhi
Printed at : Salasar Imaging System, Delhi

Dedicated To

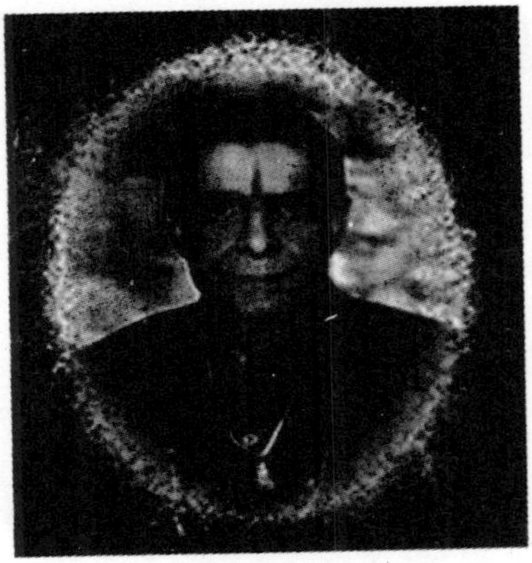

Slimming Techniques is lovingly dedicated to Respected Guru Dev (Dr.) Pt. Manmohan Shastri Ji of Babal (Ambala) for his constant gifts of light, life, inspirations and divine true love

Contents

Preface

Slimming Techniques is a book about a lifestyle—a way of life in which achievement of good health and vitality that begin with balanced food and right choice of exercise. Obesity can be controlled by eating selected foods of low energy density to modify day-to-day eating habits, to restrict the amount of energy consumed and to reduce the risk of surplus calories. For healthier living decreases in fat consumption and an increase in the consumption of complex carbohydrates is advised by the experienced dieticians. This book will provide its readers practical ways to make these changes along with advice on decreasing the intake of sugars and other food products, whilst maintaining the nutritional value of diet. As such 'Slimming Techniques' will promote a style of eating for the whole family- and not just for those trying to lose weight. I will never suggest rapid weight-loss which fails to deliver long term results.

Exercise is a vital ingredients of life. Simple movements will help to get a firm grounding to maintain a woman's body slim, trim, healthy and attractive. Yoga, modern dance, gymnastic keep fit fundamental movements—the flow of message through brain, and nerves, the circulation of blood, the rhythm of breathing and movement of muscles and bones beneath the skin.

Exercise is equally important for expectant mothers, who usually spoil their figure after childbirth. I have tried to include exclusive chapters for those likely to conceive, maintain a healthy fetus during pregnancy, have a painless labour and maintain beautiful body after the delivery besides taking care of correct make-up/health techniques during periods, pregnancy and after the delivery.

Sincere gratitude for the exceptional cooperation and contributions for assisting in preparing this book to:

Dr. D. S. JASPAL
Patron/President Indian Medical Association, Haryana

Dr. RAJEEV GUPTA, MD (Radiology)
PGIMS (Rohtak)

Dr. RITA JASPAL
Senior Vice President,
IMA-Haryana

Dr. SARITA GUPTA, MD (obst & gynae)
Saket Hospital

Parvesh Handa

1

Watch Your Weight and Figure

Excess weight is a misfortune that can become a real mental burden to those afflicted with. The problem does not represent a danger to physical health, its psychological effect can also be a serious matter. Excess weight should not be regarded simply as a misfortune, the problem calls for medical attention. If you eat properly, you are unlikely to get fat. There is a reserve distribution center in our organism, hidden away in some corner of the brain that controls the accumulation and balance of the fat in our bodies. Nervous overweight is a regulatory factor on which the metabolism of fats and water would seem to depend. To define the word 'metabolism', it means simply the process within our bodies by which nutritive material is built up into living matter. The metabolism will be defined in detail in this book.

We shall also divide overweight into three categories: fatty overweight, watery overweight (or spongy overweight) and cellulite, which are very different as regards their appearance, mechanism and treatment. Fatty overweight is really 'fat and muscle' hypertrophy. It is uniformly spread, is accompanied by a large appetite and is more usual in men. Watery overweight is a matter of 'Watery fat'. It does not affect the muscles at all , is most usual over the lower half of the body, is not accompanied by any marked appetite, and is most common in women. Cellulite is a form of infiltration rather than overweight.

Fat is an unwelcome visitor in human body. There is always fat in our body. It is only when there is too much of it that we are entitled to talk of being overweight. At the same time it acts as a storeroom for our bodies and as a protective cushion. Fat makes a covering on the surface of our bodies. It is about ¼ inches thick under the lower layer of the skin and fills the gaps in the cellular spaces or subcutaneous tissue. It gives the skin appearance of fullness, and ensures suppleness of the body's movements. It is thickest in certain places, whereas in some overweight people, it forms veritable roll of fat usually appearing on the stomach, the breasts, the thighs, hips and buttocks. In normal bodies the layer of fat should not be more than a half-inch thick. If a person is overweight, the fat spreads everywhere, but will be maximum in these parts.

Fat surrounds many of our organs, even around the heart and kidney. In case of overweight, it accumulates to such an extent that it may compress, hinder its movements and cause pain, weaken the affected organ and reduces its muscular strength. Fat is especially found in stomach and in the peritoneum where numerous folds protect our abdominal organs. On the other hand, fat is rarely found around the lungs, the brain, the genital organs and the spleen.

Human body is a laboratory. Chemically, the fat in the body can come from the fat we eat. The body is able to manufacture fat out of carbon, oxygen and hydrogen, which are basic components when fats are broken down or burned. Carbonic acid and water are the normal residues when fats are broken down. Fat is the best fuel for our body, which produces calories. A fat surplus of 8% to 15%, over the normal weight must be considered as overweight. Beyond that, it is obesity. Over 30%, is extreme obesity.

The Well-shaped Woman

She should be more rounded and softer than a man. In a woman, the subcutaneous fat is usually thicker and the muscles and bones are less prominent. The connective tissues, not the muscles mould a woman's figure.

1. Her body is less bulky and more slender than a man's.

2. Her chest is narrower, thinner and less muscular.

3. Her waist is narrower, her loins and hips are fuller.

4. Her limbs are not so bulky and do not have muscular contours.

5. Her shoulders are neater and more sloping.

6. Her pelvis is lower than a man's, looks wider because of the relative narrowness of her waist and lesser development of thighs.

7. Her collarbones should stand out slightly. It is a sign of overweight if you no longer see the collarbones.

8. Her stomach should be flat.

9. Her hipbone should show through the skin, as should the edges of the lowest ribs.

10. Her lowest vertebrae should be slightly cushioned.

11. Her calves should not show the over-developed muscles (should be slim and not bulgy).

12. Her ankles must be neat, blending gently into the lower part of the calf. The joints of lower limbs, both knees and ankles should be slim.

13. Her thighs should be completely together when you stand upright.

14. Her neck should have a clean line and never be scraggy. There should be groove at the nape running up to the back of the head. This groove fills up with the layers of the fat.

15. Her face should be well filled-out.

16. Her breasts as well as buttocks should be sufficiently fat to be rounded, although not too large or they may droop.

Weight Measurement of Women Between 18 to 25

Height in Cm. *(Shoes 5 cm Heel)*	*Weight in Kg.* *Small*	*Medium*	*Large Frame*
145	42-44	44-49	47-54
150	44-47	46-52	50-57
155	46-50	49-54	52-60
160	49-53	51-57	55-63
165	52-56	54-61	59-66
170	56-60	58-65	62-70
175	59-64	62-69	68-74
180	63-67	66-72	70-79

Weight Measurement for Men From 25 and Above

155	50-54	54-59	54-64
160	54-57	56-62	60-67
165	54-60	59-65	63-71
170	60-64	63-69	67-75
175	64-68	66-73	70-79
185	71-76	74-82	77-87
190	74-79	78-86	83-93

Ideal Weight and Measurement of Bust, Waist, Hips, Thighs, Calf and Ankle

(All measurements in inches)

Height	*Bust*	*Waist*	*Hips*	*Thighs*	*Calf*	*Ankle*
60	32	22	34	19	11.5	6.5
61	33	23	34	19.5	11.5	6.5
62	33.5	23.5	34.5	20	12	7
63	34	24	35	20.5	12	7
64	34.5	24	36	21	12.5	7.5
65	35	24.5	37	22	13	7.5
66	35.5	25	37.5	22	13	7.5
67	36	25.5	38	22	13	8
68	36.5	26	38	22.5	13.5	8
69	37	27	39	23	13.5	8
70	37.5	27.5	39.5	23	14	8.5
71	38	28	40	23.5	14	8.5

Ideally, a woman should be more rounded and softer than man. In a woman, the subcutaneous fat is usually thicker and the muscles and bones are less prominent. The connective tissues, not muscles, mould a woman's figure. Her body is less bulky and more slender than a man's. In a woman, the trunk is like a vase standing on the winder pedestal of the hips.

A young woman of average height, who is not pregnant, or who is not engaged in hard physical labor requires 2300 calories a day. The requirement of calories per day per women is as below:

Women doing very light work:	1900
Teenagers:	2000
Women doing moderate work:	2000
Women during pregnancy:	2500
Women during lactation:	2900

Calorie Consumption Per Hour

Light household work:	120-130
Hard household work:	400-600
Floor sweeping:	240-300
Boating:	125-220
Swimming:	395-475
Gardening:	200-250
Dancing:	250-350
Morning walk	150
Jogging	800
Cycling, Skating and Playing:	315-375

The Warning Signals

- When fat starts accumulating on the hips and waist.
- When the buttocks get enlarged.

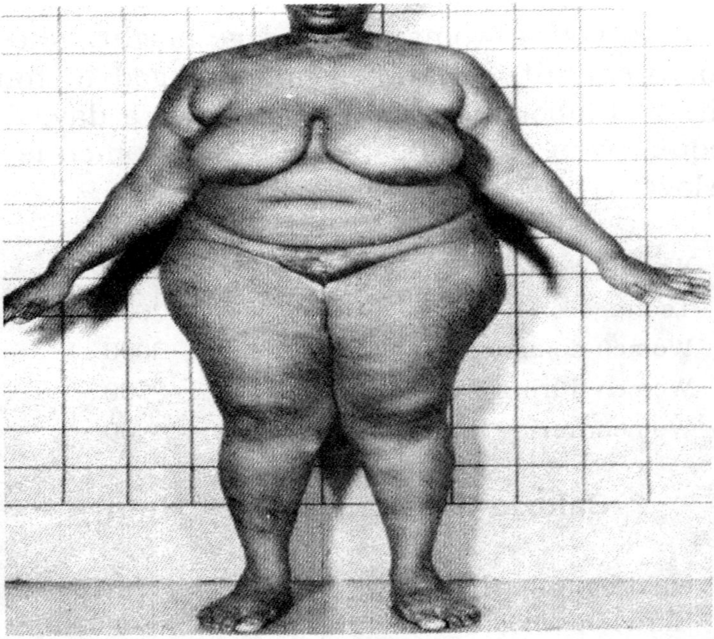

- When the neck thickens and lose its normal contour.
- When the double chin appears.
- When the skin loses its firmness and tightness.

- When the skin gets puffy.
- When the breasts begin to sag.
- When the pubis begins to swell over the genital organs.
- When the stomach muscles sag over the pubis.

Overweight Leads the Following Troubles:

- Frequent circulation trouble, as obese persons get palpitations, experience frequent pain in the heart, high blood pressure, diabetes and gout (a disease of lower joint called 'gathia').
- Psychological and Nervous trouble, which causes irritation, tiredness, nervousness, apathetic and lethargic behavior.
- Digestive trouble, which causes dilation of stomach, inflammation and spasm of intestines and congestion of the liver, fatty degeneration and digestive upsets.
- Genital disorders due to infiltration of fat into the nervous and glandular tissues, which control sexual appetite or may cause temporary impotence.

Causes of Overweight

- Heredity factor due to family tendency.
- Habit of overeating and taking too many calories.
- Ageing factor.
- Poor functioning of system.
- Nervous factors.
- Sedentary life causing constipation.
- Glandular system causing over-secretion.
- Taking excessive fat and alcohol.

Recommended Food

Food must contain a balanced quantity of proteins and carbohydrates. A young woman of average height, who is not pregnant and not engaged in hard physical labor requires 2300 calories a day. One gram protein gives four calories, whereas one gram carbohydrate also gives four calories and one gram of fat gives nine calories.

Protein is found in milk, eggs, meat, fish, soyabean, almond, coconut, groundnut, etc. Protein gives strength to the body. Carbohydrate is found in vegetables, fruits, cereals etc. It helps in digestion and also helps other foods in generating calories. Deficiency of Carbohydrates lead to weakness. Fat provides calcium to the tissues and is important for growth.

Diet Chart

	Vegetarian diet	Non-vegetarian diet
Ratio of Calorie:		
Protein	30%	30%
Carbohydrates	65%	50%
Fat	5%	20%

Food you may eat

- Non-fatty soups
- Slightly salted vegetables.
- Egg (one egg a day is sufficient).
- Fresh butter.
- Fresh or condensed milk (skimmed and unsweetened)
- Fresh cheese.
- Green vegetables and fruits
- Fruit juices and herbal teas.

Food you should avoid

- Bread, biscuit and pastries.
- Fat meats and fatty fish.
- Fried foods.
- Butter and oils.
- Cream and milk foods.
- Cornflakes, starchy flour.
- Fatty, fermented and salted cheese.
- Bananas, chestnuts, walnuts, jam, honey, cocoa and chocolates.
- Wine, beer, cider, alcoholic and sweetened drink.

Figure and Frame of Body

Girls between the age of 14 to 18 tend to put on excess weight. Measure your bust, waist and hips with a tape. Bust and hips should nearly have the same measurement. The hips should not exceed that of the bust by more than two inches. The waist should be about ten inches less than the breast. The bust should be six times and waist four times your wrist. Hips should be 6.25 times, upper thighs 31.3 times, calves 2.23 times and ankles should be 1.5 times your waist. You may compare your measurements with those given below:

- Small frame: Wrist 5-1/2 to 5-3/4 inches
- Medium frame: Wrist 5-3/4 to 6-1/2 inches
- Large frame: Wrist over 6-1/2 inches

The Daily Rhythm

Everyone's weight varies in the course of the day, depending upon what he takes in, what he gets rid of and what he uses up on exercise. Weight is at its lowest when we wake up in the morning. The difference can be only partly explained by night losses. Meals increase weight temporarily. They give rise to increased nutritional exchanges, and bring about a sudden fall in weight. The fall partly compensates for the additional weight of the meal. If we don't eat enough, this stimulation of nutritional exchanges ends up in an actual loss of weight. Two things make you slim. They are: complete rest for watery overweight and intense sweaty exercise for fatty overweight. Moderate physical exercise is effective against cellulite, which indicate three conclusions:

1. Meals and excretions have less effect on daily weight than is generally supposed.

2. Weight usually increases towards the evening.

3. The night's rest largely supplements the part played by night losses in causing one's weight to be at its minimum in the morning.

The factors such as meals, excretions and exercises are not the only factors. There are the effects of emotion, irritation and nervous fatigue those bring about losses or gains in weight.

The Monthly Rhythm

Women have normal fluctuations in weight especially during the time of their periods. Women should weigh themselves only once a month on a definite day. Their weight begins to increase in the three days immediately before the onset of their period. The weight further increases when the periods start. During this time they often feel thirsty. This weight is kept up, because of less urination during the period, then falls and returns to its usual level within three to four days after the end of the menstrual flow.

Along with the weight the hip, midriff and waist measurements increase by half-an-inch to an inch as the period approaches, which corrects itself after the period is over. These increases result from additional water being carried in the subcutaneous tissues at the time of the menstrual period.

The Balanced Diet

Eating sensibly is not easy these days as our generation is obessed with the so-called fast food culture. A balanced diet should include fruits and vegetables. These are not only rich source of vitamins and mineral salts but are also fiber-rich foods. The fiber-rich diet helps our digestive system and makes heart strong. The diet should be low in saturated fats (fatty substances that melt only in high heat and boost weight gain) and are rich in fruits, vegetables and fibers. Vegetables should form 15 to 25% of daily intake, followed by fruits about 10 to 15%, then dairy products and meats, which should be not more than 10% each. Fats, oils and sweets should not be over 5% in daily diet. Intake of six to eight glasses of water every day are must. Water flushes out the toxins from the body, keeps the skin cells hydrated and helps in keeping youthful and cheerful lessening the signs of ageing. Switching to vegetable unsaturated oils is better to our overall health. Excess of salt ends up in water retention. Substitute sugar by 'gur', jaggery and honey, is beneficial as they are compounded with vitamins and minerals.

The calcium requirement in human body increases with the advancing age. Therefore, at least two glasses of milk consumed daily are must after the age of 40. Include products like curd, cheese, eggs and fish in your daily diet. What you eat affects your health, appearance, personality and performance. The nutrients in food supply the body with energy and ensure proper body functions. Vitamin supplements should be taken under doctor's guidance as overdose of certain vitamins can lead to toxicity. Remember, overweight people need to change their lifestyles not just their diets. Many medicines can cause weight gain, several others stimulate appetite and a few alter metabolism.

2

Controlling Your Weight and Body

Are you one of those who always worry about your weight? Is it hard for you to maintain a normal figure? Two Thousand Five Hundred years ago Hippocrates – the father of medicine noted that "fat men die all of a sudden". This is true, sudden death occurs so often in fat people. People who are sluggish are steadily gaining weight. In other words, *the longer your waist line, the shorter your lifeline.* It is very important to watch your weight, not allowing yourself to become too thin or too fat, but remain near the ideal.

Changes often come on in the late twenties, reducing a person's physical fitness. Sluggish habits begin to develop as the individual loses his/her skill in running, swimming, or other healthy activities. Yet in spite of warnings from nature, they continue to eat heartily, adding many unnecessary kilos and finally losing their athletic figure and unattractive appearance.

Most of plump people give all manner of excuses for their fatness. But in almost every case the only reason is that they are eating more than they themselves really need. In other words, *extra weight is due to extra eating.* It is surprising, just a few extra calories a day will affect youthful looking appearance. For instance, if you take just one extra slice of bread a day above your actual needs and continue this for five years, you will add over 20 kg. to your figure and in ten years you will gain weight above 40 kg. Remember, all this extra fats puts a strain on your heart, kidneys and liver, and also on the large weight-bearing joints such as hips, knees and ankles. This means your body is wearing out more rapidly, carrying round all this extra weight. Those excess calories in your diet can be deadly. *You are shortening your life at your own dining table.*

Your Ideal Weight

What is your ideal weight? That depends on your height, sex, age and the type of body. There are different standards for men and women, and for people with large, medium and small frames. You may refer the height-weight measurement table in Chapter 1 in this book. People with large bones and well-developed muscles may seem somewhat overweight compared with those of lighter build. But actually the lighter persons may be carrying around more fat. His muscles may be weak and under-developed.

What should you do? First of all, try to find out why you weigh so much more than you should. Some people are overweight because they are worried and frustrated. Munching adds weight rapidly. If a person is gaining weight, it means he is taking in more calories that he is using. How many calories do you need per day? That depends on the number of things, such as the kind of work you are doing, your age, your body build and how active you are. A hard-working laborer may require 5000 calories a day. To keep going he should need only 2000 calories a day. An housewife busy around the house all day, may need 2500 calories. But an office secretary may do well on 1800 calories a day. It all depends on how active we are. At about 25 years of age, one usually burns up calories without any difficulty. At 35 the situation begins to change, one is now less active. This means, we must gauge the amount of food according to the work we do. Other major conditions that affect a person's weight are water accumulating in the tissues under the skin and overeating. Either, we must increase the output of work or we must reduce the food intake. For instance, a failing heart may produce marked swelling in the legs and other parts of the body.

How to Lose Weight Without Tears?

Dieting is not new to most people who are overweight. Usually, they have all tried this many times before. They practice to go without food entirely for a short time, only to return again to their former habits of overeating. The only solution is a completely new pattern of living outlined below:

Take Smaller Quantities of Food: Continue with a balanced diet. Quality, not quantity, is the rule. Be sure to include reasonable amounts of potatoes and whole-grain cereals in your diet. Eating slowly will help. Avoid all foods that are oily or high in fat.

Be Careful About 'Leftovers': Many housewives put on weight because they hate to see food wasted. Far better to prepare less food and avoid the problem of 'leftovers'.

Stop Nibbling Between Meals: Train yourself to get along on less food. Soon you will enjoy living on a reduced diet.

Sensible Exercise: Such exercises taken every day will help to use up those extra calories. The best exercise is walking, helps putting those large leg muscles to work, will burn up unwanted calories.

Avoid Rich Desserts: All that excess sugar and fat is high in calories but low in food value. Your best exercise is to push yourself away from the dining table while you are still hungry. Stay away from ice cream, pastry, rich cakes and sweets.

Regular Eating: Remember, regular eating is important. Your meals should be smaller than average, well-prepared and attractively arranged on the table to enjoy your meal.

Do Not Go Hungry for Long: Eat regularly but sparingly is the best way to reduce weight.

Be Sure to Have a Good Breakfast: This will carry you through the day, and you will be less tempted to nibble sweets and snacks between meals.

Use These Foods Freely: Green leafy vegetables, tomatoes and carrots — they all are low in calories, but high in vitamins and minerals and have real food value. They can also be used to ward off hunger between meals.

Overweight people tend to suffer from serious conditions, such as high blood pressure, shortness of breath, sleeplessness, heart trouble, kidney disease, diabetes and disorders of the liver. Bringing the weight down to normal will help the heart and every other organ in the body. Watch for high calorie/ low calorie foods as detailed below

High Calorie Foods

Cashew nut (per 100 gm of edible portion)		596 calories
Coconut	-do-	661 calories
Cake, Chocolate	-do-	400 calories
Butter	-do-	729 calories
Ghee fresh	-do-	818 calories
Vegetable cooking oil	-do-	900 calories
Ice cream	one small cup	150 calories

Low Calories Foods

Cow's milk	(per 100 gm)	67 cals.
Curds	-do-	46 cals.
Buttermilk	-do-	15 cals
Orange	-do-	53 cals.
Banana	-do-	100 cals
Leafy vegetables	-do-	13-90 cals.

How to gain weight?

If you are a little under the normal weight, you have certain advantages in health. Thin people often live longer, provided they are not suffering from some wasting disease such as tuberculosis. But if you are very much underweight, you ought to at least have a complete medical examination to be sure there is nothing seriously wrong inside.

There are two types of thin people. One type is wiry and energetic. Such people are seldom sick. They eat heartily, but never put on weight because they probably burn up their energy. Most of such people like to put on weight for the sake of appearance. The other types of thin people are not wiry and energetic. They lack energy and drive. Most of them tired easily and their own digestive organs are unable to digest even normal meals. Rich foods usually make them feel sick. Some people have small stomach with low capacity and help themselves by taking smaller meals and eating more frequently. They should choose plain but rich foods.

Low weight people should have a complete X-ray of the digestive organs to rule out the possibility of some hidden disease. A stool test is advisable to check possibility of worms, amoebic infection and other harmful parasites. A complete blood count is recommended to be sure there is no anemia. The urine should also be carefully checked to eliminate any infection in the kidney or bladder. Nervous anxiety is another cause of anorexia or lack of appetite. The child or a woman who feels rejected may suffer from a chronic type of anxiety in which he never seems to have a normal appetite. A few multi-vitamin tablets help to increase the appetite and return the body's functions to normal. The following treatments are suggested to gain weight and relieve nervous strain:

1. Avoid taking snacks just before meal, which often spoils the appetite.

2. Eat a well-balanced meal, keeping on a high calorie-diet as much as possible.

3. Avoid use of tobacco, particularly just before meals.

4. Learn to relax; this will help reduce nervous tension while bringing the body's activities back to normal.

5. A quiet rest just before the dinner and also after lunch may be all needed to bring back life and vitality to the whole body.

6. Cut down on all extra activities; this will help to reduce tension.

How to Grow Taller?

Normal growth is an amazing process. From the moment of conception until the day a baby is born, growth is extremely rapid in womb. After birth, the baby continues to grow rapidly for the first two years, then the process of growth begins to slow down. Once again around the age of 13th or 14th year, a rapid growth begins. This is the time known as adolescence. Girls grow more rapidly than boys because their hormones are more active in early puberty. Later the boys catch up and overtake girls, usually reaching their full height between the 16th and 19th years.

A person's height depends to a large extent on the length of the long bones in his lower extremities, particularly the femur in the thigh and the tibia in the leg. For good stature, the spinal bones or vertebrae must also be well developed in proportion to these long bones. Near the end of the bones there is a transverse area known as the epiphysial line consisting cartilage in which the young bone cells are growing. During childhood and youth these young bone cells are continually adding to the length of the bones. This is how there is gain in height and weight.

Hormone Changes

The thyroid glands may often alter a person's height. In hypothyroidism there is delay in growth and development along with some mental slowness, fatigue and also menstrual disorders. Hereditary factors always play a large part in body development. Growth failure in children may be due to severe factors, such as:

1. Child's diet may be lacking in essential nutrients (vitamins, minerals and protein).

2. Certain diseases involving organs such as the liver, kidneys, pancreas, heart or lungs may all contribute to a failure of normal growth.

3. Foods may not be properly absorbed and utilized by the body.

4. Congenital heart disease must be considered when the growth is subnormal during childhood or youth.

5. Thyroid deficiency may result in cretinism and hypogonadism, both of which retard normal growth.

Consult a doctor to find the possible cause of the growth failure. Females with this condition are given estrogenic substances. A diet rich in protein and minerals is valuable. If a tumor is present in the pituitary, X-ray therapy or surgical removal is the treatment of choice.

3

Slim 'n' Trim by Exercise

Physical Culture for Beginners

Several exercises have been described for slimming and developing the muscles of each and every part of the human anatomy in this chapter. The checking of measurement should not be taken weekly or even monthly as only disappointment will be felt. Once every thirteen weeks is quite sufficient. A standard measurement is given below as a guide:

Date ____

____

Height_______ft.________in Weight(kg)______________

Reach_______ft.________in. Neck______________

Chest(Contracted)__________ Expanded______________

Waist__________________ Hips______________

Forearm________________ Biceps________________

Wrist________________ Thighs________________

Calf________________ Ankle________________

Physical Culture for Beginners

1. Exercises should be performed in open air, or at least in a well-ventilated room, and clothing should be of lightest description-shorts for preference.

2. Concentration is also of the greatest importance. Close the eyes and visualize the particular muscle or set of muscles affected becoming larger and stronger while contracted. Do not allow the mind to wander during exercise. Superb muscular development depends upon the complete concentration of the muscles, followed by their complete relaxation.

3. Breathing must be through the nose — on no account should the mouth be used for breathing. All the exercises must be performed slowly and without jerkiness.

4. Exercise of muscles: Hold the particular muscle or set of muscles should be contracted with vigor for a second or two. The exercises may be repeated a certain

number of times until the muscles become slightly tired. Fatigue must be avoided.

5. The best time for exercise is in the early morning before one's bath and never within an hour of a meal.

6. Give the muscles a rest on one day in the week, the benefit is apparent the following day.

7. Exercise with the feeling and intention that the body shall benefit.

8. In summer or in tropical countries, coarse wheaten-meal should take the place of oatmeal, as the latter is too heating. In olden times this was not so, as the flour mills were then stone mills.

9. The ideal form of diet, however, should consist of five parts of Carbohydrates to one each of Albumin (such as meat, fish, eggs, milk, cheese, peas, beans etc) and Fat (such as butter, oil, egg-yolk, nuts etc.) with the addition of a liberal supply of raw fresh fruit and vegetables in the form of salads.

10. Foods, which requires cooking in a fireproof glass casserole, so as to conserve the vitamins. Fresh food, which contains vitamins should always be preferred to

canned, frozen or other preserved food. Full-corn bread is also a preventive of constipation. Use brown sugar in preference to white. Don't eat polished rice. Potatoes should be boiled, baked or roasted in their skins.

11. Growing children should be given cod-liver oil. After exercise in the morning, drink a glass of pure cold water, and about six glasses during the day. After early morning glass of water, eat either an apple or an orange, or begin breakfast with raw fresh fruit.

12. Dress: Wear air-mesh underclothing in winter and summer. Do not wear tight-fitting clothing nor tight-fitting shoes. One should not overload oneself with heavy clothing.

13. Bathing: Take a daily bath after exercise and before breakfast. Take a cold shower, a warm bath should be taken once a week just before going to bed.

14. Sun bathing: Should not be indulged in by those of a nervous temperament or who have or are suspected to have had the tuberculosis, without the approval of a doctor. Commence with an exposure of ten minutes, then gradually increase the period.

15. Walking: Next to swimming, walking is one of the best form of exercise. Do not carry the chest in a constrained position, but keep the head up and the back of neck pressed against the collar. Keep the shoulder blades in and do not allow them to protrude as if they were embryonic wings. The legs should swing from the hips, and each arm from the shoulder in unison with the opposite leg. Land on the heel and take off on the toe. Eight hours sleep daily in a room where fresh air circulates and be examined carefully by a qualified doctor once a year are Golden Rules.

Exercises for Slimming and Development of Muscles of Body

Exercise to rejuvenate body

Lie full length on the back, knees straight, heels together, feet pointed, arms on the ground

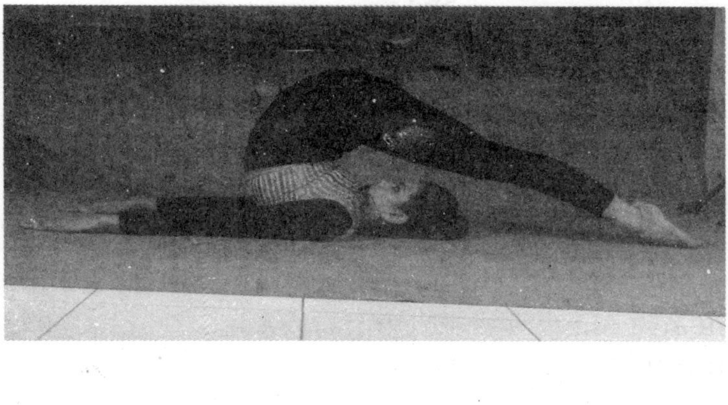

by the sides and palms downwards. Bring legs slowly upwards above the head keeping knees straight, heels together and touching the ground lightly behind the head. Hold. Return to the initial position. Repeat three to four times.

Developing the Muscles of Neck

Lie down full length on the back, feet together, knees straight. Raise the arms and take to the point of the chin between the forefingers and thumb of each hand. Now raise head from the ground, at the same time press down with both hands. Hold for some time. Lower the head

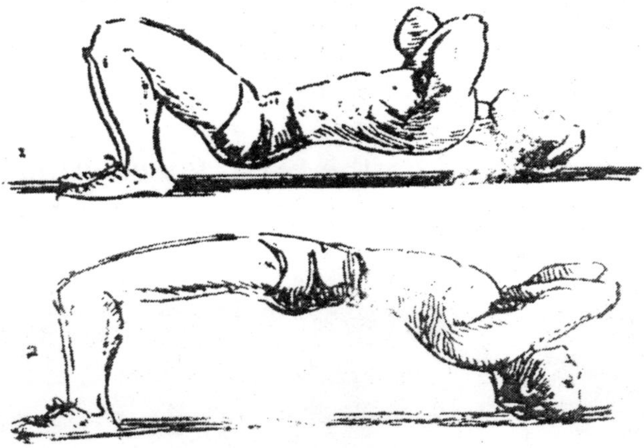

to the ground still maintaining the pressure with hands. Exhale as the head is raised, inhale as head is lowered. During the exercise concentrate the mind on the muscles in front of the neck.

Here is another exercise to strengthen the muscles of neck. Lie on the back, knees bent, feet planted firmly on the ground and apart. Raise the back and shoulders from the ground so that the weight of body is supported on the feet and back of head. Hold. Lean back slowly so that the weight of the body is transferred from the back to the front of head. At the same time allow the folded arms to drop backwards and above the face. Hold. Repeat without allowing the back or shoulders to touch the ground. Use a small cushion placed under the head while exercising.

Inhale as the weight of the body is being transferred from the back to the front of the head. Exhale as the weight is being transferred to the back of the head. Concentrate the mind on the muscles at the back of the neck.

Developing the Muscles of Shoulders

Stand erect with heels together and toes turned outwards. Keep knees straight. Clench the fists tightly having backs of the hands to the front.

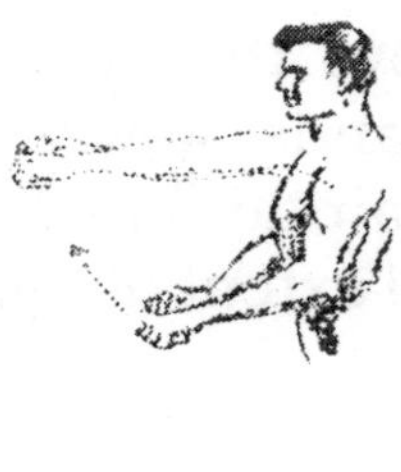

Raise arms in front to the level of the shoulder exerting strong pressure downwards. Lower the arms alternatively on left and then on right sides. Relax. Inhale as the arms are raised, exhale as the arms are lowered. During the exercise concentrate the mind on the contracted muscles of the shoulder and chest

Developing the Muscles of Upper Portion of Back

Stand erect with the heels together, toes turned outward, knees straight. Grip the hands

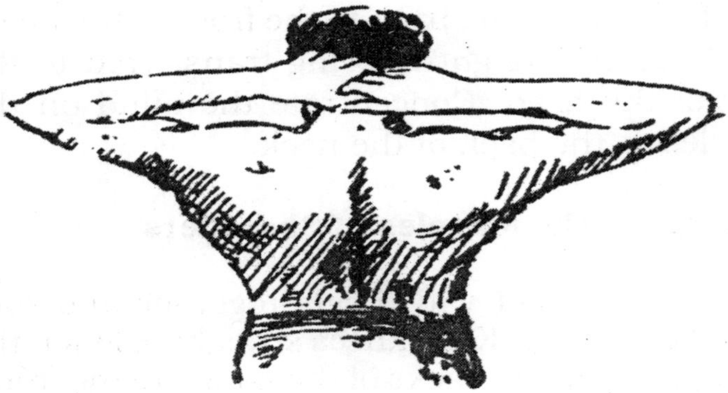

at the full extent above the head pulling them strongly. Lower the hands slowly to the back of the head. Hold. Still maintaining the pull of raised hands slowly to the full extent of the arms, change the grip of the hands. On completion of the exercise drop the arms to the sides and relax. Inhale as the hands are raised, exhale as the hands are lowered. Concentrate the mind on the contracted muscles of the upper portion of the back.

Stimulating the Upper Back and Ribs

Stand erect with heels together. Raise the arms laterally, grip the hands above the head, look upwards and pull the hands strongly. Hold. Now lower the arms laterally contracting the muscle under the arms. Grip the hands at the full extent of the arms behind the back. Hold. Repeat. On completion of the exercise drop the

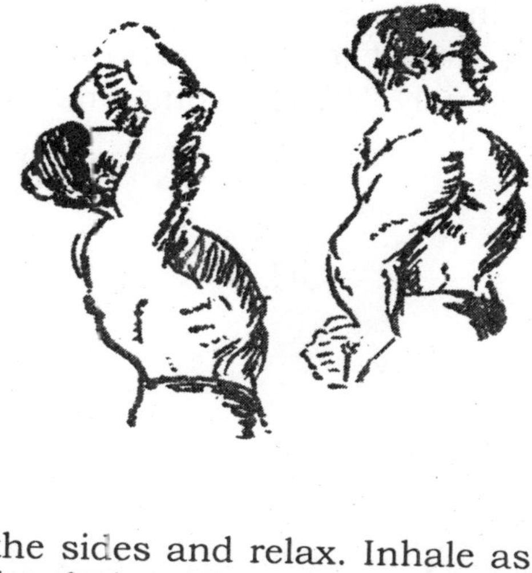

arms to the sides and relax. Inhale as the arms are raised, exhale as the arms are lowered. During the exercise concentrate the mind on the contracted muscles of the back, ribs and shoulders

Developing Abdominal Muscles

Lie full length on the back, hands clasped under the head, knees straight, heels raised slightly from the ground. Now raise the right leg

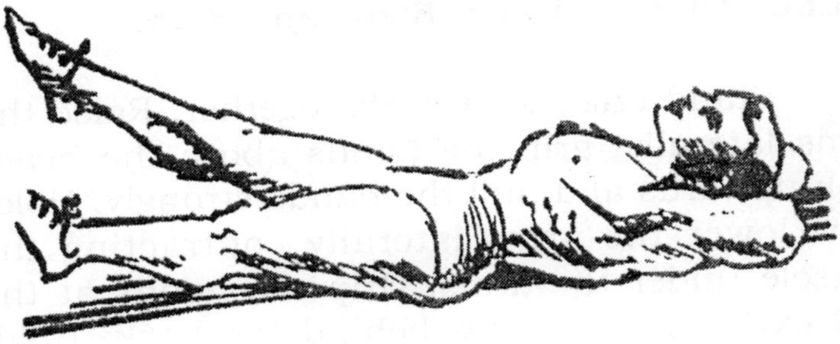

slowly, keeping the knee straight. Slowly lower the right leg almost to the ground and raise left leg simultaneously. Hold for some time and repeat

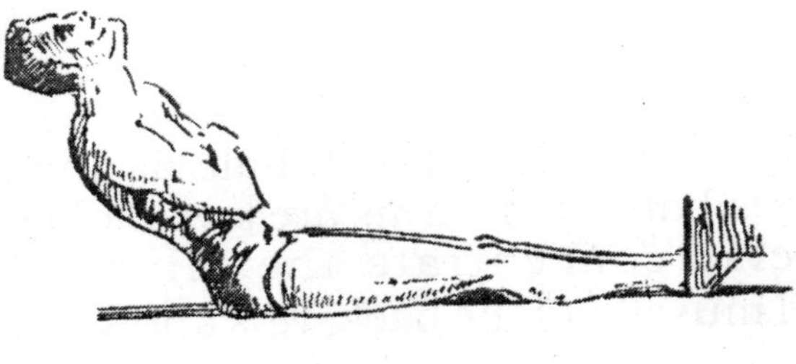

exercise on other leg. On completion of the exercise, relax by lying with the arms on the ground. Exhale as the leg is raised and inhale as the leg is lowered. During exercise concentrate the mind on the contracted abdominal muscles.

Here is another exercise to develop muscles of the abdomen. Sit down on the ground with feet in front. Lean slowly backwards and touch the back of the head lightly on the ground. Rise slowly to a sitting position, strongly contracting the muscles of abdomen. Inhale as the head and body are lowered, exhale as the body is raised. During the exercise concentrate the mind on the contracted abdominal muscles.

Slimming the Trunk

Stand erect with feet apart, knees straight and body evenly balanced on both feet. Raise the arms laterally outwards from the sides until they

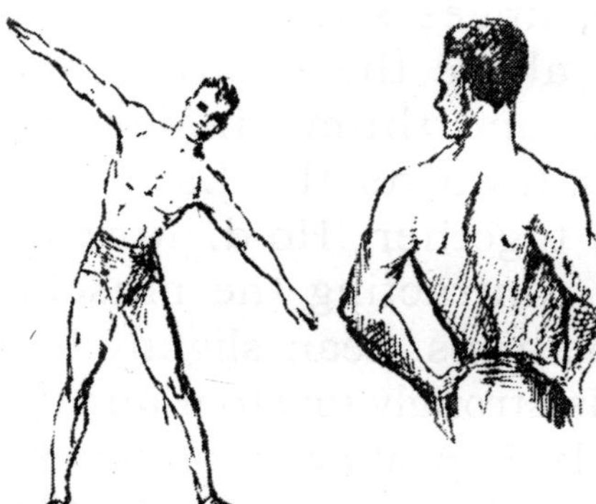

are on a level with the shoulders. Keep the legs straight and knees braced, bend the trunk to the left contracting the muscles on that side. Hold. Repeat exercise on other side. Now drop the arms to the sides. Repeat four to five times. Exhale during the bending of the trunk, inhale while resuming the position. During the exercise concentrate the mind on the contracted muscle of the sides of the trunk.

Here is another exercise for slimming and strengthening the muscles of the sides of the trunk. Stand erect, feet apart, knees straight, body evenly balanced on both feet. Place the hands on the hips, heels of the hands pressed well down, elbows backwards. Turn the trunk slowly round to the left as far as possible. Repeat by turning right and left alternately. On completion of the exercise drop the arms to the sides and relax.

Developing the Muscles of the Chest

Stand erect, heels together, toes turned outward, knees straight. Now raise the arms laterally above the head, bringing the hands together, one thumb inside the other. Look upwards towards the hand and press them strongly together. Hold. Now lower the arms laterally contracting the muscles of the chest under the arms. Lean slightly forward, pressing the hands strongly together one thumb inside the other. Hold. Repeat five to six times. On completion of exercise drop the arms to the sides. Relax.

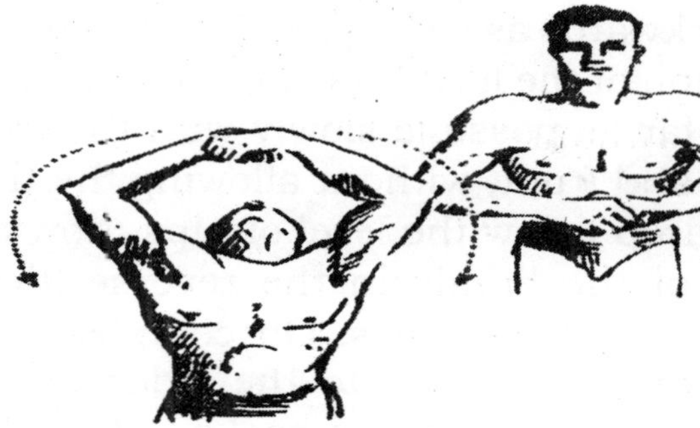

Inhale as the arms are raised, exhale as the arms are lowered. During the exercise concentrate the mind on the contracted muscles of the chest and upper ribs.

Stimulating the Waist and the Digestive Functions

Stand erect, feet apart, knees straight. Grip the hands behind the head and pull them

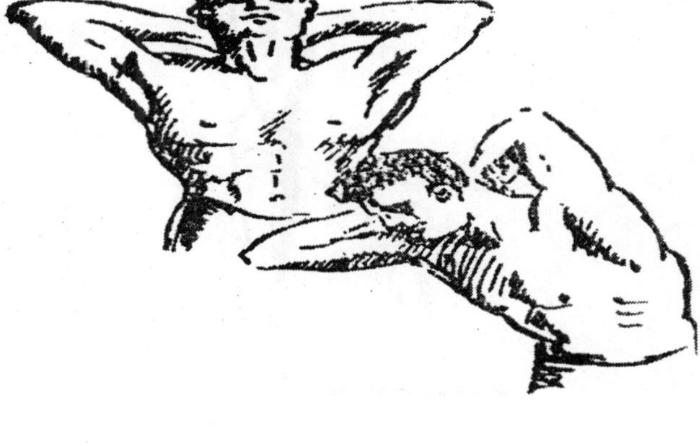

strongly. At the same time lean the head and trunk backwards as far as possible without altering the position of the feet, legs and hips. Have a large circle as far as possible slowly with the trunk on the right and front, without allowing the trunk or arms to drop below the level of hips. Now change the grip of the hands in the reverse direction. Repeat six to eight times. On completion of the exercise drop the arms to the sides and relax. Inhale as the trunk circles backwards, exhale as the trunk circles to the front.

Exercise to Relieve Extra Fat on the Back

Stand erect, feet apart, knees straight, body evenly balanced on both feet. Raise the arms to the full extent above the head. Keeping the knees braced and the legs steady, lower the trunk

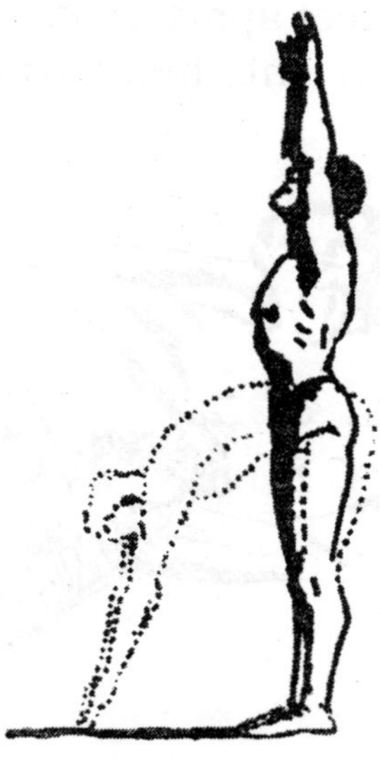

stretching the hands as far to the front as possible, and touch the front of the feet. Now raise the trunk still stretching the hands as far to the front as possible. Then lean back as far as possible without altering the position of the legs. Hold. Repeat. On completion of the exercise drop the arms to the sides and relax. Inhale as the trunk is raised, exhale when lowered. Concentrate the mind on contracted muscles.

To Slim Heavy Thighs

Stand erect, heels together, knees straight. Bring right leg to the front, knees straight, turn the toes upwards, pressing the heels down as far as possible, thereby contracting the muscles on the front of the leg. Hold. Then bend knees and bring the leg to the rear thereby contracting the

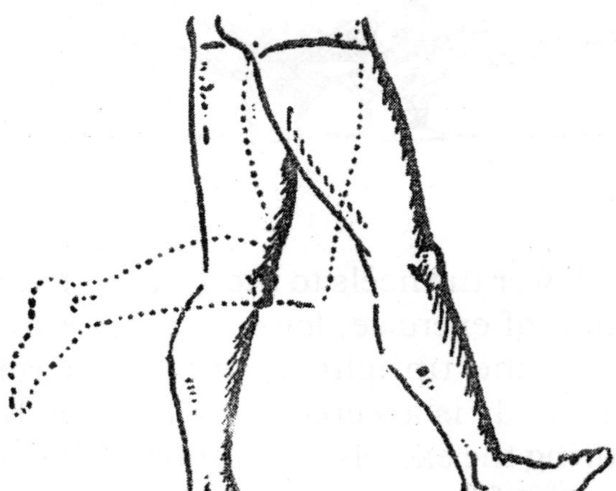

muscles of the back of leg. Hold. Continue and repeat with the left leg. On completion of the exercise, resume the upright position and relax. Breathe normal and concentrate the mind on the muscles on the front of thighs.

Developing Thighs, Hips and Calves

Stand erect, heels together, toes turned outwards, knees straight. Clasp the hands behind the head. Rise on the toes and sink slowly downwards. Hold. Rise slowly to the upright

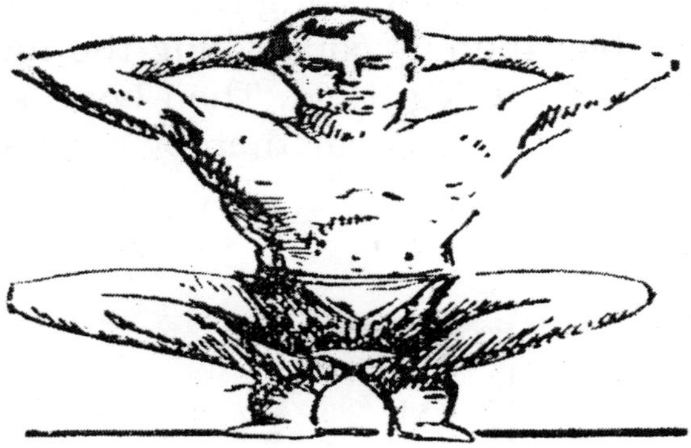

position and lower the heels to the ground. Repeat. On completion of exercise, lower the arms to the sides, resume the upright position and relax. Exhale as the body is lowered, inhale as the body is raised. During the exercise concentrate the mind on the muscles of the calves and the front of the thighs.

Developing the Muscles of Spine

Stand upright, heels together, toes turned outwards, knees straight. Lean the head forward and clasp the hands behind the head, without exerting any pull. Raise the head upwards and backwards, at the same time pulling strongly downwards and forwards with the hands, thereby contracting the muscles on either side of the upper part of the spine. Hold, and repeat. Lower the arms when exercise is complete. Inhale as the head is raised, exhale as the head is lowered. Concentrate the mind on the contracted muscles.

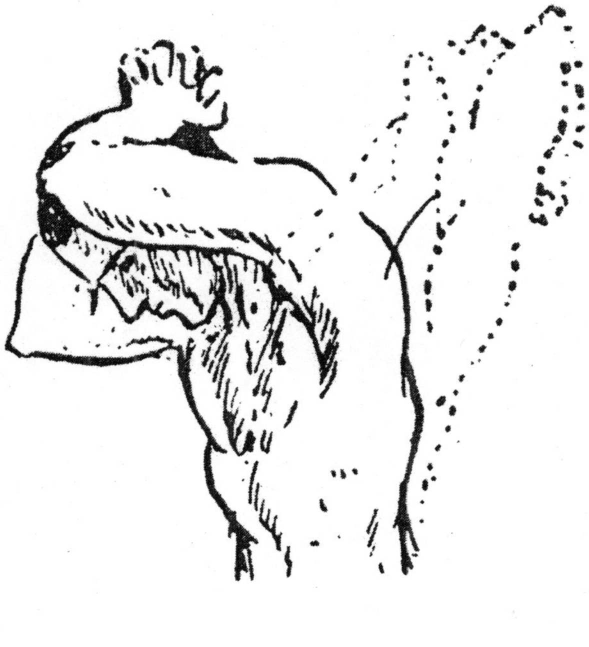

4

Overweight

A fat surplus of 8% to 15%, over the normal weight, must be considered as overweight. Beyond that, it is obesity. Over 30%, it is extreme obesity. Overweight not only affects your looks, but your health too. Beware of overweight, it causes:

Circulation Troubles

The obese person gets palpitations, experiences pains in the heart. Moreover, the heart itself gets tired because it is burden by the fat surrounding it and the very substance of the heart muscle is impregnated. The heart trouble is generally associated with arteriosclerosis and high blood pressure possibly with diabetes or gout.

Psychological and Nervous Troubles

These are common afflictions amongst obese people. The obese people are subject to nervous instability. Get rid of surplus flat and you will probably regain your calm and balance.

Digestive Troubles

They are usually the result of the intemperance of the obese, rather than of their weight. Dilation of the stomach, painful digestion, inflammation and spasms of the intestines and congestion of the liver can be accounted for in this way.

Genital Disorders

Genital disorders are the dominating factor in the mind of those persons suffering from obesity, particularly where men are concerned. The infiltration of fat into the nervous and glandular tissues, which control sexual appetite and can cause impotence. This may be only temporary, but if it is felt too long the cells may mortify. When slimming, taken in time, they will regain their vitality and sexual desire will return. For both men and women, sexual troubles disappear under treatment and the glands regain their vitality. This is especially so in the case of woman who thinks she is sterile, but after slimming finds she is pregnant. The low intensity of menstrual flow or even its disappearance could have caused her to make this mistake.

Fatty Overweight

This is found particularly in men. The increase in weight is spread uniformly over the whole body. It is often noticeable over the upper half of the body (head, neck, arms and trunk) than on the lower limbs. There is both an excess of fat and over-development of muscles. This is not really solely fatty overweight. It could be called "energetic overweight". The dangers, which threaten such people include cholesterol, gout, stones, hypertension, coronary thrombosis, diabetes etc.

The Causes.........

Due to heredity factor: Often there is family tendency to stoutness, which is more often the inheritance of the habit of overeating rather than a truly genetic factor.

The age factor: Some people who have been able to eat excessively with impunity up to a certain age, find that when with age they become dangerously obese. This may be caused due to poorer functioning of the system.

Due to overeating: Excess weight in relation to the size is the result of taking in too many calories with food and consequently building up a reserve in the form of an overdeveloped layer of fat, usually due to inability to control a large appetite.

The part played by a sedentary life: This is the logical complement of overeating. If we store up fattening substances, it is not only because of absorbing too much but also because we are using up relatively too little by not taking enough muscular exercise.

Part played by nervous factors

The effect of your glands: When fatty overweight is accompanied by glandular symptoms, when in the majority of cases the latter are the effects and not the cause. They usually disappear when the obesity is cured. In this type of overweight, however, over- secretion of sub-renal glands play a major role.

How to Treat Fatty Overweight?

Above all, reduce your intake of food thereby reducing the amount of fat put to reserve. The following treatments are suggested to combat overweight:

Dieting : This is very essential part of the treatment. What is needed is a quantity diet on

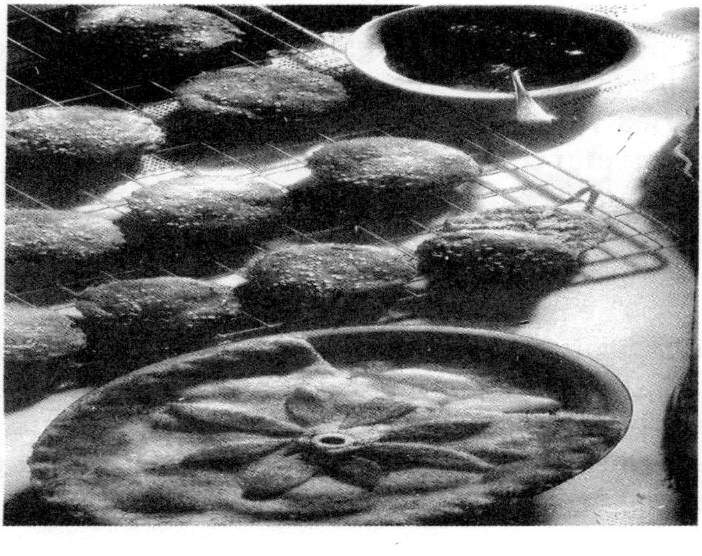

the one hand and a quality diet on the other. The first thing to do is to lower the number of calories taken daily to about 1300 to 1600 calories every 24 hours. Cut out fat and alcohol. Reduce carbohydrates to a minimum, but retain a sufficient amount of protein for your own needs.

The Food You May Eat

1. Non-fatty soups, vegetable broths without bread and slightly salted.
2. Mutton, lean fish, lean poultry — without sauce or butter.
3. Egg (one a day).
4. Small quantities of fresh butter and liquid paraffin.
5. Fresh or condensed milk (skimmed and unsweetened).
6. Fresh cheese with low fat contents.
7. Potatoes in very small quantity.
8. All green vegetables and fruits.
9. Salt in very small quantity.
10. Fruit juices, herbal teas and light wines. Never drink when you are eating.

The Food You May Not Eat

1. Bread, biscuit, pastries and jam.
2. Fatty soups, fat meats and fatty fish.
3. Meat in sauces and stews.
4. Fat pork meats.
5. Fried foods.
6. Lard, margarine, butter, oil, cream and milk products.
7. Cornflakes, starch, flour and rice.
8. Fatty, fermented and salted cheese.
9. Dried vegetables and mushrooms.
10. Bananas, chestnuts, walnuts, jam, syrup, honey, cocoa and chocolate.
11. Wine, beer, cider and all kinds of alcoholic or sweetened drinks.

Exercises and Gymnastics

1. Take energetic exercise: physical training, gymnastics exercises and sports of all kinds. If you are really obese you must wait until dieting has slimmed you down.

2. Gentle activities, such as walking, promote assimilation and therefore added weight, are not recommended.

To Eliminate Excess Water

There are various ways of 'sucking out' a large amount of water in order to eliminate it. The first, by drugs, consists of purging. This causes water to be absorbed into the intestines. The second consists of the use of diuretics. And the third is sudation and sweating.

Use of Drugs

When you are on strict diet, the discomfort of hunger can be minimized by drugs. But these drugs are not to be used when the patient is not a big eater or if he/she can control appetite without too much difficulty. These appetite reducing 'psychamines' are available in pill form. These drugs may cause fewer secondary complications, such as insomnia and palpitations. These drugs, like many others, if taken uninterruptedly, prove habit-forming. You may avoid this by going without them for ten days every month and relying on your will-power during that time to avoid any success. Your doctor will take advantage of this pause to increase your urinary output by means of diuretic drugs. Heart sufferers must avoid taking such drugs.There drugs can cause damage if not taken correctly on proper medical advise.

Psychological Treatment

Emotional shock can be a cause of overweight. This must be fought by personal determination. However, Psychamine drugs can be of great assistance. Consult a doctor in case you are unable to control the disorder.

Hydro-thermal Treatment

These are recommended as a useful auxiliary means of getting rid of superfluous weight.

You are fat-prone, If

- You like to eat very well-and do.
- You have rather sedentary habits or a sedentary job.
- You put on weight during holidays.
- Emotional upsets and worry make you lose weight.
- Massage and douches have little effect.
- Sweating session cause moderate but lasting loss of weight.
- Cutting down on your food has a noticeable effect.

- Overweight has overtaken you at a time other than at a stage of sexual development, such as puberty, menopause, pregnancy.

- The overweight affects the upper part of the body, such as arms, shoulders and face as much as or more than the lower part.

- Overweight is accompanied by circulation trouble.

- You rarely feel cold.

What You Should Do?

- Weigh yourself every 28 days.

- Cut down on your food, and cut out, in particular, biscuits, bread, cakes.

- Use little salt and no sugar.

- Breakfast on tea and apples.

- Don't drink, while you are eating.

- If necessary, reduce your appetite by taking psychamines an hour before meals.

- Take Foam Bath or Turkish Bath.

- Have 20 minutes of physical exercises preceded by muscular limbering up, every morning and energetic sports.

- Drink diuretic water.

You Must Never

- Weigh yourself very frequently.

- Lose patience.

- Let yourself become constipated and take drugs of your own accord without consulting a doctor.

5

Watery Overweight

Watery overweight is one of the commonest form of female overweight. It is almost exclusively female described as spongy obesity. The main characteristic of this type of overweight is that it is paradoxical obsity. It is infact a unique syndrome characterised by retention of fat and water together. The main characteristic of this type of overweight is that it is paradoxical. It cannot be explained by overeating.

Symptoms of Watery Overweight

This type of excess weight occurs almost solely in women, sometimes in young women, but more often still in young girl who is just entering the early years of adulthood. It may also occur at the menopause. The odd thing about this type of excess weight is that it affects the upper limbs and the chest relatively little. Rather it predominates over the lower half of the body, the hips and the buttocks. From there, it extends to the stomach, the thighs and the inside of the knees. The patient complains of cold feet and hands, which appear red and damp. Often chilblains occur, even in summer. Moreover, red blotches appear on the legs, which increase in size, begin to get rough, coarse-grained, veined and stiff. They hurt when they are touched. The patient complains of a frequently twisted ankle. The nails break or split.

In nearly all cases of watery overweight, irregular and painful periods among women, intestinal swelling, a painful tension in the chest and nervousness are the common symptoms. In most of the cases, periods last only two or three days and are accompanied by headaches.

Causes of Watery Overweight

1. *Food*: Dieting will be an important part of the treatment. However, overeating does not usually account for overweight at all. This lack of balance in feeding — with too much water not enough albumin — leads to stopping the normal chemical reactions through its alkalizing character, and seems to prevent our body getting rid of the surplus water, which then accumulates in the tissues.

2. *Salt*: Also plays a significant part. Salt holds water. At the beginning of menstruation the blood becomes loaded with salt, which explains the retention of water usual at this time. In order to combat the retention of

water and thirst, we must strictly limit the intake of salt.

3. *Exercise*: Plays an important part. It is absolutely contra-indicated here, as is walking or gymnastics. It causes you to put on weight, whereas rest and lying down reduce weight considerably.

4. *Age*: It is also very important. Paradoxical overweight occurs especially at the time of sexual development and change. A woman can expect an improvement with marriage and her first pregnancy. At the menopause, a woman can expect her circulatory condition to become stable.

5. *Endocrine factors*: It is in fact a matter of phases of sexual development rather than age. Retention of water in the tissues, owing to decrease in urinary elimination, is encouraged, not only by lack of balance in food intake, but also by ovarian or pituitary activity. Normal women usually gain a little weight (about 500 gms) when their period starts, and lose that when it is over. In case of watery overweight, this loss does not occur. So the woman puts on weight successively and each monthly period. Estrogenic hormones increase this overweight in women, and induce abnormal retention of water. Watery overweight often occurs at a stage of sexual development,

such as puberty, pregnancy, miscarriage, a natural or induced menopause.

6. *Psychological factors*: The emotional element can often effects severe mental shock.

7. *The electro-chemical balance of the body fluids*: It is the electro-chemical balance of the blood and of the resulting lymphatic fluids. There is evidence, in cases of watery overweight, of a deficiency in the blood of some metallic catalytic agents (such as zinc, copper, nickel, manganese or perhaps cobalt) varying from one patient to another. Treatment by giving very small doses of these metals results in favorable changes in the electrical charges of the different elements in the blood, thereby preventing certain abnormal chemical activities.

The Treatment of Watery Overweight

Diet : Unbalanced eating is in the origin of this kind of overweight. Dieting is the leading factor in its treatment. Dieting will follow these general principles:

1. Never drink with your meals and drink very little between meals.

2. Don't salt your food.

3. Few vegetables and plenty of meats (in case of non-vegetarian).

4. No watery foods, such as soup, juicy fruits, melon etc.

(**Note**: Get medical advice before embarking on strict diets).

Rest: Exercise, overwork, walking, fatigue and late nights encourage overweight. You must relax and rest. Good results are achieved from resting in bed. A lying down position causes an increase in urination. Cases are known of young women regularly losing 5 to 7 kg a week during three weeks in bed.

General Massage: Reflex therapeutic massage acts indirectly by its effect on nervous system and by the relaxation it brings.

Get Rid of Water by Sweating, Laxatives and Diuretics:

Paradoxically, these are ineffective in cases of watery overweight. They cannot bring about a permanent loss of weight in case of pure watery overweight, as there is no surplus fat to break down. This is why sweating, laxatives and diuretics are of no use. The only solution is gradually to reduce this abnormal need of the tissues for water by cutting down water intake over a long period, by diminishing the intake of salt and by taking on the electro-chemical balance of the blood.

You Have Watery Overweight, If:

- You eat moderately. Putting yourself on a vegetable and fruit diet and even cutting down your food considerably.
- You overstrain yourself physically and mentally.
- You take rest and relax, which are immediately beneficial.
- Emotion and worry cause you to put on weight.
- You don't feel really well.
- Sweating cause temporary loss of weight.
- You have serious trouble with your periods which sometimes diminish or disappear altogether.
- The overweight occurs at the time of a change in sexual development.
- The overweight is predominantly in the lower part of the body, on hips, buttocks and thighs.

- You have serious circulation troubles when legs are veined, dry and rough, and the ankles are heavy and swollen by the evening.
- You have chilblains every winter.
- Your nails split.

What To Do?

- Weigh yourself every 28 days.
- Cut out bread and cakes. Avoid vegetables, juicy fruits and soups. Eat eggs, meat and cheese (unsalted).
- For breakfast eat an egg, cheese or yogurt.
- Don't eat and drink at the same time. Drink very little between meals.
- Rest and relax as much as possible.
- Drink mineral waters, which encourage total elimination.

What You Must Not Do?

- Weigh yourself constantly.
- Lose patience.

- Go without food, or cut out meat and put yourself on vegetables and fruit exclusively.
- Indulge in physical exercise and exhausting sport.
- Go to bed late.
- Take strong purgatives.
- Get constipated.
- Take drugs without medical supervision.
- Follow a dry diet without medical supervision.

6

Cellulitis

The essential difference between cellulite and fatty obesity or watery obesity is that it affects certain limited areas on body only, whereas fat and water invade large areas on the body. A woman with cellulite may have it only on the hips or the nape of her neck, or in both legs, the rest of the body being unaffected.

What is Cellulite?

Cellulite is an inflammation of the connective tissue caused by poisons accumulating there instead of being thrown out by the body. The most common of these poisons are uric, lastic and oxalic acids. In case of cellulite, the double chin, thick shoulders and swollen ankles are stuffed with organic waste matter, which is normally rejected through urine, sweat and bowels. This waste matter often collects in the connective tissue.

The connective tissue is to be found in the body wherever there are no organs. Under the skin, it is known as subcutaneous cellular tissue. In case of cellulite, this connective tissue fills with lymph containing much waste matter, which irritates and causes it to contract. It then fills with water, which the body is prompt to supply in order to dilute the poisoned lymph and relieve the irritation of the tissues. Water thickens into mucus, which in turn becomes semi-solid matter. This congests the cellular tissue, which then becomes painful. This is cellulite. Cellulite is not exclusive to women. Nearly 30% of cases afflict men.

How to Diagnose Cellulite?

Cellulite begins on the inside surface of the thighs and knees, covering up the bone projections. It quickly moves down to thicken ankles, which disappear from view. This thickening becomes more and more pronounced and soon affects the whole leg from the ankle to the knee. Gradually but relentlessly, over the months and years, the thickening of lower limbs continues and the sides of the thighs swell out in their turn. The hips become heavy with rolls of fat and affect the buttocks and rest of body, which include the thick neck, swollen napes and heavy shoulders.

At first, the tissues have a soft consistency and are not painful. Sometimes, it is difficult to distinguish from watery or fatty infiltration. Later, pinching the skin is painful and may produce small wrinkles. Cellulite may be suspected from the badly nourished appearance of the skin rough, grayish and cold. At the stage of confirmed cellulite, the symptoms are clear when the skin give a feeling of padding. The skin adheres to the underlying tissues, instead of making for suppleness and become inflamed. The pinching is usually painful and causes bruising. At the atrophy stage, you will feel underneath the skin small balls or little grains: a kind of nodule, which rolls around under your fingers.

The Organs Attacked by Cellulite

- The inside surface of the thighs
- The knees
- The ankles
- The hips
- The nape of the neck
- The back of arms
- The shoulder- blades and spinal column
- On the forehead and lower part of the face.

The Dangers Due to Cellulite

Cellulite overweight does not bring the organic disorders caused by obesity. You can die from obesity, you will not die of cellulite. More serious cellulite will give rise to nervous pressure resulting in severe pains, occurring more often at night giving rise to insomnia, which contributes to the disorder of the nervous system.

Factors Causing Cellulite and the Treatment

Heredity, feeding (a cellulite mother often have a cellulite daughter), abnormal activity of the liver generally due to dieting and sedentariness are some of the factors favoring cellulite. To burn up toxins in the body exercise your muscles. Toxins can be burnt up only by oxygen. Oxygen can consumes poisons at only two points: the lungs and the muscles, which work together for purification in the body. Fatigue, like sedentariness is a important factor in cellulite and these can be relieved by regular exercising, but avoid over-exerting your body. Learn to breathe in open air. Remember, kidneys do not render poisons harmless, their job is to spot them and throw them out of body. Avoid poisonous foods and alcohol that attack three basic defences — the digestive system, the nervous system and the kidney system. For the treatment of cellulite following steps are advised:

Dieting

Have judicious eating with low calorie content. Good food should make up for the normal wear and tear on our tissues. Ban everything which is highly seasoned – condiments, spices, salt and pepper or toxic such as coffee, tea, alcohol, tobacco, highly fermented cheese or too acid – tomatoes, lemons and over-cooked foods such as stews, fatty pork meats, sauces, cooked butter and fried foods. A cellulitic should avoid as much as possible oily fish certain meats, some of the vegetables (broad beans, split peas, soya), all dried fruits, milk products, tobacco, confectionery, all spicy things (mustard, pickles, garlic) and drinks (all alcoholic drinks, coffee and tea)and tobacco. Eat meals at regular hours (do not eat between meals). Try hard to eat in peace, away from noise and completely relaxed during meals. A cellulitic will need only a cooling diet, rich in green vegetables and well-balanced menus.

Exercise

Physical exercise plays a part in burning up poisons. So if you are going to stop the body fluids becoming clogged, you must make sure that you exercise your muscles sufficiently. But too violent exercise resulting in fatigue, increases the poisoning of the system and has precisely the opposite effect of what we want. Cellulitic need plenty of fresh air (open air walking) and active muscular life. For how long you should walk or have exercise, there is no single rule for everybody – each has own staying power and resistance. The length of walk cr exercise may be increased from five minutes the first day to half-an-hour after a week, 45 minutes after a fortnight, half an hour twice a day after three weeks. Do no wear high-heeled shoes.

Rest

It is not only immoderate physical exercise that cause strain. Everyday life (pure simple and the harassed life) causes it too. Remember, the body substance and nerve centers have to be restored at regular intervals and need periodic rest. If your working life is already exhausting, don't add to it extra strain. Generally speaking, eight hours' sleep is essential for people who use up a lot of energy. The ideal is to go to bed at 10 p.m. and get up at 6 a.m.

Breathing

Breathing in burning up the poisons in the blood is equally important, as oxygen is the great purifier of the bloodstream. Lungs, too, need all the vital forces in the atmosphere, which come from the sun, the earth and are breathed out by every living thing, such as flowers, birds and trees. We must find fresh air. We must shun stuffy atmospheres and crowded streets as much because of our need for this vital force the oxygen. Start breathing in gently, first inflating the upper part of the thorax, and moving the arms to the horizontal and then slightly backwards. The complete breathing in process should take 6 to 12 seconds. Breathing out should be done slowly. Begin by collapsing the upper part of the chest, then the lower part, and end by contracting the stomach. To empty the chest completely, lower the arms, the shoulders and the head being bent slightly forward and back slightly arched.

Massage

Gentle and gradually increasing massage, which arouses sensation rather than pain and always dispel cellulite from the place to which it is applied. Various massage movements applied on body will be described in detail in one of the coming chapter. Remember, massage should never cause pain, but should be hard enough all the same to arouse more sensitivity than it would have done on a perfectly healthy area.

The best time for massage is in the morning, when the inflammation of the cellulite tissue is at its minimum. Cellulite is always more evident in the evening because of fatigue. Morning massage can be deeper, hence more effective. Do the massage three times a week, about 35 minutes each time, having draining for 5 minutes, roll-massage for 5 minutes, rapid massage on all the least affected areas for 10 minutes, direct massage on most painful areas for 10 minutes and general draining movements for 5 minutes. Finish with a cold shower and friction with a loofah or a rough towel. You will be able to recognize good and effective massage by the fact that the ganglions (of the groins for the legs, of the armpits for the arms) have enlarged and do not hurt after the session. If the massage is too violent, the ganglions will not enlarge until the next day and will be painful.

Remember, It Is Cellulite, If:

1. It is localized and begins on the inside surface of the thighs and knees.

2. The skin is in-filtrated, padded and has the elastic consistency of a sheet of rubber.

3. The skin is not mobile, it cannot be squeezed and develops the "orange peel" look.

4. The skin hurts when touched.

5. Bruises appear very easily.

What To Do in Case of Cellulite?

1. Take regular, well-balanced meals with low calorie content.

2. Daily exercise, not too energetic. Open-air walking and light sports are very beneficial.

3. Rest as often as possible; relax.

4. Breathe efficiently, with your chest and with your stomach.

5. Massage yourself on right principles without causing pain or discomfort.

6. Increase the intensity of the massage progressively, but never let it become painful.

7. Before and after the massage, do drainage movements in the direction of lymphatic circulation.

What You Must Never Do?

1. Do intensive physical exercise.

2. Start massaging vigorously right away, thereby causing discomfort.

3. Get bruised after massage.

4. Get tired and stiff after walking.

5. Eat indigestible foods.

6. Drink alcoholic drinks.

7. Smoking.

8. Drinking too much coffee or tea.

9. Live in stuffy atmosphere.

10. Exhaust your nerves too much.

11. Regularly attend badly ventilated and smoky public places.

Obesity

Obesity and overweight complaints are quite common. There are several causes for obesity; majority of the causes are due to overeating and lack of exercise. The logical way to lose weight is to cut down food intake by 100% without affecting the nutritive value of the food consumed and exercise regularly to burn the extra fat.

1 kg of body fat contains 7500 kcal energy. If you reduce 250 kcal from regular food intake and burn another 250 kcal by exercise - the total calorie reduction amount to 500 kcal or roughly 3500 kcal per week. Thus the total reduction in weight per month will be 2 kg. This is considered to be the safe method of losing weight. All weight watchers should keep in mind the following tips to lose weight till desired limit is reached and to maintain thereafter:

1. Fast for longer period (10 to 12 days under the supervision of an expert).

2. Reduce butter, fat, fried foods, cheese, cream, soups, cakes, sweets and sugar.

3. Avoid cakes, pastries, biscuits and salted nuts. Use only skimmed milk.

4. Stop alcohol. Eat more watery vegetables and fruits to subside the appetite.

5. Do not eat without knowing the calories value of the food.

7

Metabolism and Recommended Dietary Allowance

Anatomy and Physiology

To achieve self-grooming, it is essential to have thorough knowledge of the working of human body and major body systems to explore its specific structures i.e. anatomy and functions. The major body systems include:

1. Integumentary System
2. Skeletal System
3. Muscular System
4. Respiratory System
5. Circulatory System

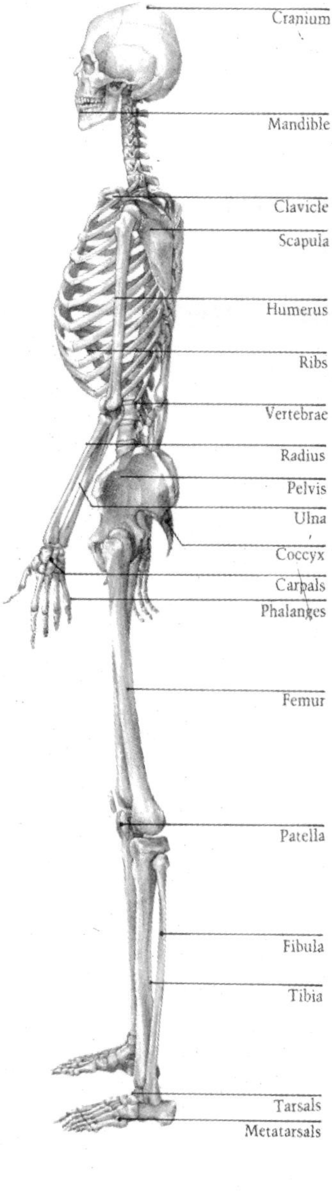
Cranium
Mandible
Clavicle
Scapula
Humerus
Ribs
Vertebrae
Radius
Pelvis
Ulna
Coccyx
Carpals
Phalanges
Femur
Patella
Fibula
Tibia
Tarsals
Metatarsals

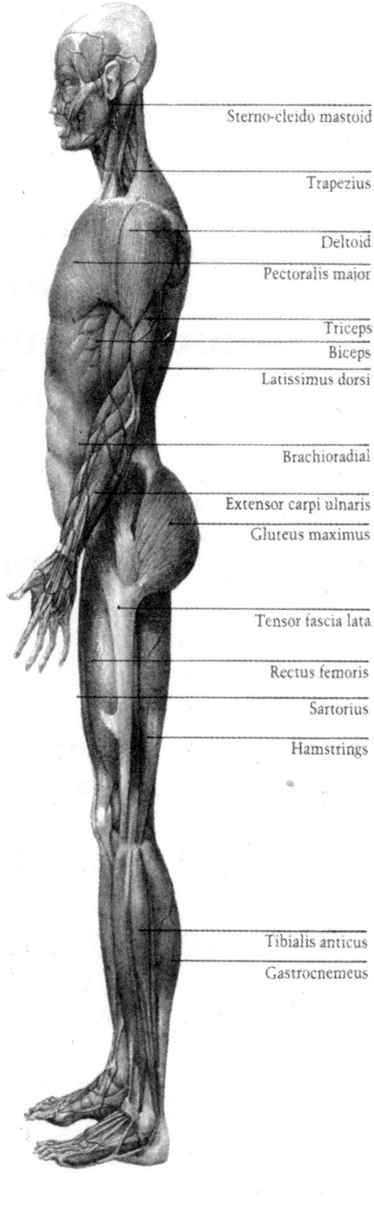
Sterno-cleido mastoid
Trapezius
Deltoid
Pectoralis major
Triceps
Biceps
Latissimus dorsi
Brachioradial
Extensor carpi ulnaris
Gluteus maximus
Tensor fascia lata
Rectus femoris
Sartorius
Hamstrings
Tibialis anticus
Gastrocnemeus

6. Digestive System

7. Genito-Urinary System

8. Nervous System

9. Endocrine System

The Cells

The human organism is made up of a vast variety of parts that vary in complexity. These include organ systems, organs, tissues and cells. The cell is the basic structure from which all other body structures are made. These are the basic units of all living things, including bacteria, plants and animals. The human body is composed entirely of cells, fluid and cellular products. Cells are made up of protoplasm — a colorless, jelly-like substance in which food elements such as protein, fats, carbohydrates, mineral salts and water are present. Cells have the following principle parts:

1. Cytoplasm: Found outside of the nucleus and contains materials necessary for the growth, reproduction and self-repair of the cell.

2. Centrosome: It is a small, round body in the cytoplasm, which also affects the reproduction of the cell.

3. Nucleus: A small spherical body composed mostly of ribonucleic acid (RNA) and the protein within the cell nucleus. It plays an important part in the reproduction of the cell.

4. Cell membrane: It encloses the protoplasm and permits soluble substance to enter and leave the cell.

Growth of Cell

As long as the cell receives an adequate supply of food, oxygen and water, eliminates waste products and is favored with proper temperature, it will continue to grow and thrive. However, in case these conditions do not exist and there is the presence of toxins (poison) or pressure, then the growth and the health of the cells are impaired. When the cells reaches maturity, reproduction takes place by direct or indirect division. Direct division (Amitosis) is a simple process whereby the cell elongates. His method of reproduction occurs among bacteria and plant life but rarely takes place in human tissues.

Indirect division (Mitosis) is a complex process whereby a series of changes occur in the nucleus and this method of reproduction occurs in human tissues.

Metabolism

A chemical process in which, the cells are nourished and supplied with energy to carry on many activities in human body. In a healthy body, the metabolic rate is kept under control by a secretion from the thyroid gland. There are two phases of metabolism:

Anabolism

A constructive process which build up larger molecules from smaller ones. During this process the body stores water, food and oxygen for the time when these substances are needed for cell growth and repair.

Catabolism

An destructive process, which breaks down larger substances or molecules into smaller ones. This process releases energy that can be stored by special molecules to be used for muscle contraction, secretion or heat production.

Both Anabolism and Catabolism are carried out simultaneously in the cells so that their activities are closely regulated and balanced with building up and energy consumption. However, if we use less energy than we manufacture, we may notice a weight gain. If molecules of energy are not used, they turn to fat. To get rid of built up fat, more energy-usually in the shape of exercise, must be used or less energy through food taken in.

The cell in a human body is a minute part that makes up each of the individual systems. The

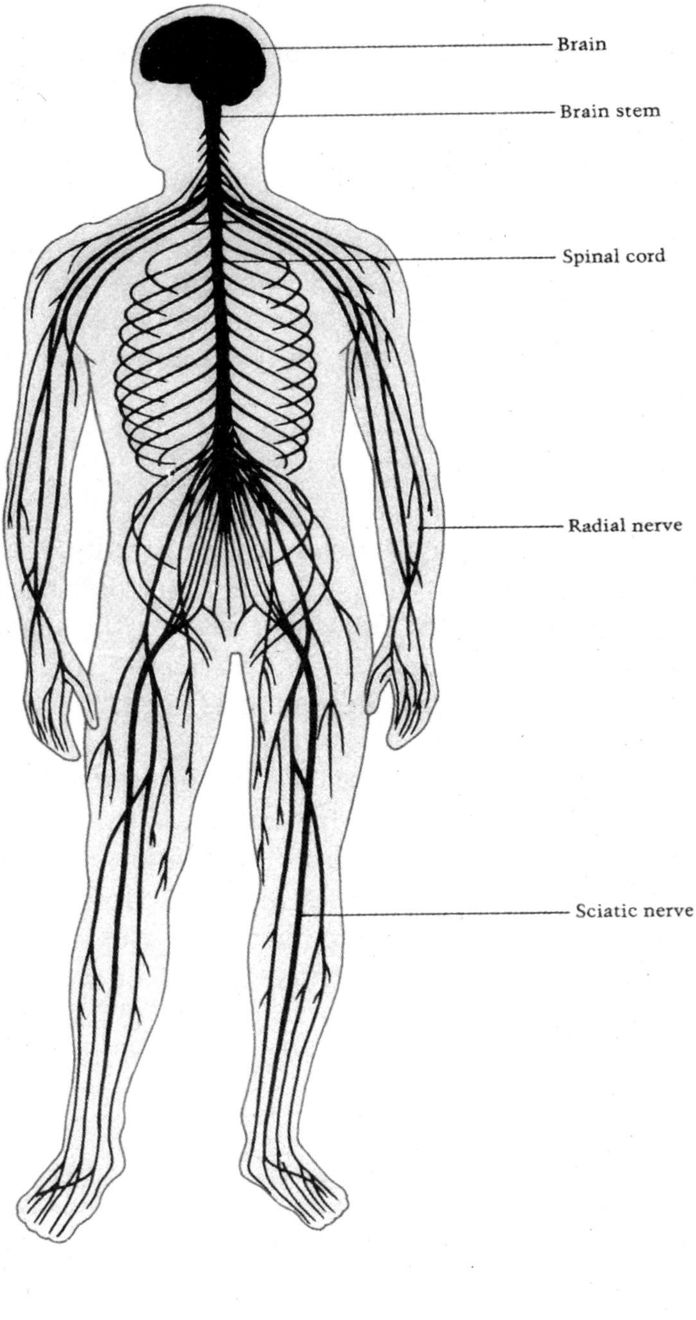
Brain
Brain stem
Spinal cord
Radial nerve
Sciatic nerve

body is made up of millions of individual tiny microscopic cells. They are built into tissue, organs and glands, body systems and finally the human organism. The cells varying in size and shape are made of protoplasm — a colorless, transparent, jelly-like substance consisting of nearly 70% water together with organic and inorganic substances.

Body Tissues and Organs

Tissues are composed of group of cells. Each tissue has a specific function and can be recognized by its characteristic appearance. They are of five types:

1. Connective tissue (Fat tissues): Serves to support, protect and bind together tissues of the body.

2. Muscular tissue: Contracts and move various parts of the body.

3. Nerve tissue: Controls and coordinate all body functions.

4. Epithelial tissue: A protective covering on the body surface, such as skin, mucous, membranes, linings of heart, digestive and respiratory organs and glands.

5. Liquid tissue: Carry food, waste products and hormones by means of the blood and lymph.

Organs

Organs are structures designed to accomplish a definite function. The important organs of the body are:

1. The brain: which control the body.

2. The heart: which circulates the blood.

3. The lungs: which supply oxygen to the blood and control respiratory system in the body.

4. The liver: which removes toxic products of digestion.

5. The kidney: which excrete water and other waste products.

6. The stomach and intestines: which digest the food.

Body Regions

The skeleton is divided into three main regions: the skull, the spine and the limbs. Respiration is the controlled exchange of gases – oxygen and carbon dioxide by the cell to activate and energy needed for the cell to function. The blood carries oxygen from the respiratory system and nutrients from the digestive system to the cells and are absorbed through the cell membrane by diffusion, osmosis, dissolution, active transport and filtration.

Role of Metabolism

Metabolism is series of chemical reaction, which utilizes the nutrients for growth, repair or energy production within the body. The metabolism is the rate of which the body uses energy for the process of metabolism. The energy is measured in kilocalories (kcal) or kilojoules. One calorie is the amount of energy required to raise the temperature of 1 kg of water by 1 degree C. The joule is the metric unit of measurement for heat and energy (1 kcal : 4.2 kj) The graph below shows energy value of nutrients.

Nutrients	**Energy value**	
Carbohydrates	3.75 kcal	[16 kj]
Protein	4.00 kcal	[17 kj]
Fat	9.00 kcal	[37 kj]

Energy Requirements

The amount of food, which a person requires depend on the energy used each day. This varies according to age, sex, body structure, occupation, physical activities and the conditions such as pregnancy or health. In fact, ideally the food eaten each day should supply no more and no less than the amount of energy used in that day. The average energy requirements for an adult woman is approximately 1940 kcal and for a man 2550 kcal. Occupations are classified according to how active they are, as following:

Sedentary: Office workers, clerical tasks, teachers and shop workers.

Moderate active: Hairdressers, beauticians and postman.

Very active: Construction laborer, athletes and hockey/football players.

Leisure activities: Jogging.

Special needs: Extra energy is required during the final months of pregnancy and breastfeeding.

Basal Metabolism Rate (BMR)

This is amount of energy required to keep the body alive when it is warm and at complete rest. It is used to keep the heart, lungs and digestive system moving in maintained brain., functioning of the body and all chemical reactions in the body. Women tend to have a lower BMR than men because they are lighter and have less muscle tissue. The BMR is also lower in elderly people and during periods of starvations, when the body needs lower food energy.

The average values of BMR for person aged 40 year are:

Women: 1360 kcal (5700 kj) per day.
Men: 1750 kcal (7300 kj) per day.

As an example the table below illustrate the energy used for various activities (25 year old office worker weighing 62 kg)

Activity	*Kcal/hour*	*kj used/hour*
Sleeping	57	238
Sitting (eating)	66	300
Standing (cooking)	126	540
Washing and dressing	126	540
Walking moderately quickly	210	900
Walking up/down stairs	390	1680
Office sitting	90	360
Office walking	156	660
Dancing	270	1140
Average jogging	390	1620

In case of the following conditions, seek advise of a doctor:

- If the age is under 18 or over 70 years.
- Undergoing medical treatments.
- Severe obesity.
- On a medical prescribed diet.
- Pregnancy or feeding a child.

Dietary Advice for Weight Loss

1. The best way to lose weight is to combine a diet with an exercise program.
2. Aim for a small, steady weight loss of half or one kg per week.
3. Avoid crash diets.
4. Other than a reduction in energy content, the diet must be well balanced.
5. Eat at least three meals a day, so that energy intake is spread evenly.
6. Try to avoid eating in between meals.
7. Drink plenty of fluids.
8. Include treats, occasionally as reward.

Recommended Dietary Allowance

The recommended dietary allowance (RDA) suggests for Indian men and women the major nutrients usually required by men, women, working women, lactating mothers, and during pregnancy. An adult woman should consume approximately 1900 to 2200 and a man approximately 2200 to 2500 kcal/day as daily energy requirement. However, during pregnancy and breastfeeding energy requirement are higher and a woman needs between 2200 to 2500 kcal/ day. These requirements should be supplemented by a balanced combination of carbohydrates, protein, vegetables and fat moderation. The keyword here is quality and not quantity. It's not how much you eat but what you eat. The following tips are suggested. However, all food groups provide energy, which is expressed in technical terms as kilocalories (kcal):

- Protein (65 gm/day): is required for a good overall growth and development. Pulses, dairy products, soyabean are excellent sources of vegetarian protein.

- Calcium (1000 mg/day): is required for the development of bones and teeth. Dairy products, soybean products, green leafy vegetables and sesame seeds are loaded with calcium.

- Iron (40 mg/day): is essential component of hemoglobin that supplies oxygen to each cell of human body (required for the production of red blood cells). Foods with high iron sources are dried beans, cereals and pulses, dried fruits and green leafy vegetables.

- Folic Acid (400 mcg/day): is a essential vitamin required especially for women going to conceive and also during the early stage of pregnancy for the growth of fetus and during pregnancy and breastfeeding. Its deficiency leads to anemia. Potatoes, vegetables, cereals and pulses, soyabean, nuts and sesame seeds are rich source of Folic Acid.

- Fat (30 gm/day): is essential to enhance energy.

- Vitamin C (40 mg/day): is necessary to fight against infections and diseases. It provides structure to bones, cartilage, muscles and blood vessels. Citrus fruits, amla and vegetables boost up plenty of vitamin C.

- Vitamin A (Beta-Carotene 2400 mcg/day): is required for clear vision and healthy skin. Excessive vitamin A leads to toxicity and can be harmful. Vitamin A level can be maintained with yellow orange, vegetables (carrot and pumpkin), fruits (mango, papaya, and tomatoes), green leafy vegetables and whole milk.

- Vitamin D: is synthesized through sunlight, aids the absorption of calcium in body.

8

Diet and Nutrition for Weight Loss

Good health largely depends on the Nutrition. To sustain life and perform various functions, men need a wide range of nutrition including proteins, fats, carbohydrates, vitamins and minerals. These are the chemical substances derived from the food. The food we eat daily, classified as cereals, pulses, legumes, nuts, oil seeds, vegetables, fruits, milk and milk products. Food in general is grouped into two nutritive, which provide energy, heat and nutrition. Non-nutritive provide only energy vitamins and minerals, which play a very important role in the regulation of metabolic activities. Minerals are useful in the formation of body structure and skeleton.

Carbohydrates

Provide energy to the body and help control break down of proteins and protect it from toxins even to burn the fat, the basic presence at carbohydrate is very essential. Glucose is the basic chemical that provides energy to the body. These are simple sugars, which get easily converted into energy. Complex carbohydrates are generally found in cereals, grains, vegetables and fruits. Since complex carbohydrates take a longer time to digest than the simple ones, they are more effective in controlling hunger.

Proteins

These are various combinations of essential Amino Acids. To maintain life and promote growth protein is very essential. Complete protein keep one alive, but do not support growth. The dietary proteins are broken down into amino acids and absorbed as such and the body synthesis them again into proteins as and when required. All foods, except refined sugar, oil and fats contain some quantity of protein in varying degrees. Milk, oilseeds, nuts, pulses and soyabean contain a good amount of protein. Proteins are required for maintaining the wear and tear of the tissue in adults, for growth in infants and children, for fetal development during pregnancy and milk generation during lactation. An adult requires protein to the extent at 0.7 gm/kg of the body weight if the quality of protein is good. The requirement should be 1 gm/kg of body weight if one takes a mixed vegetable diet. Children during growing age require slightly more proteins than adults.

Fat

Fat is an essential part in body, but if taken in excess is harmful to the body. Fat generally breaks up in the absence of carbohydrates to provide energy. Since fat is a concentrated source of energy, any excess intake of fat accumulation is termed as obesity. The fat we eat consists of fatty acid. Fat is very important for absorbing vitamin A D E and K. The body needs fat for growth and repair. The fat accumulated in the tissue give shape and cushioning effect to the body and acts as an insulator fat which helps in regulating body temperature. The most important aspect of dietary fat is its degree of the saturation. The higher the saturation, the greater the chances of accumulation of cholesterol in the body,which leads to heart diseases. In India, people generally consume regularly about 40-50% of calories as fat. Eating too much fat make one obese because each gram of fat yield twice the amount of energy produced by carbohydrates and proteins.

Fibre

There are two kinds of fibre : *soluble and insoluble.* Fibre is the non-digestible part of the plant food which consists of mainly complex carbohydrates. Fibre is generally found in whole grains, fruits and vegetables. Soluble fibre is found in oat bran, rice bran, rolled oats, carrot and pectine, beans and 'methi'. Soluble fibre increases excretion of cholesterol and also regulates blood glucose levels by delaying absorption of carbohydrates. Insoluble fibre increases the bulk of stool and substantially reduces the time taken for food to pass through intestine. The increase in bulk relieves constipation as food travels faster through the intestines and is less exposed to toxins.

Calorie Content

The calorie is a measurement of energy content in food. We need energy from food to live and carry out our daily activities and when we eat more than the energy required, the excess energy is stored in the body as fat. So we become overweight. To stay slim and healthy, we should balance the energy input with the energy output. The chart given below may be used to check the approximate calorie content of food we eat every day.

Recipe/ Cereals/ Rice/ Bread/ Noodles		*Calorie Value*
Plain Rice (cooked)	100 gm.	175
Curd Rice	100 gm.	250
Chapati	20 gm	70
Paratha Plain	each	150
Paratha Stuffed	each	200
Dosa Plain	each	150
Masala Dosa	each	200

(Contd.)

(Contd.Table)

Recipe/ Cereals/ Rice/ Bread/ Noodles		*Calorie Value*
Puri	each	95
Bread Plain	2 slices	154
Brown Bread	each (20 gm.)	40
Toast with butter	each	100
Samosa (medium size)	each	100
Idli	each of 45 gm.	100
Vada Sambar	2 no.	140
Baked Masala Puri	each of 75 gm.	188
Baked Noodles	100 gm	175
Dokla (steamed)	each of 35 gm.	35
Soyabean Tikki	each of 45 gm.	125
Fresh Maize Tikki	each of 45 gm.	110
Cabbage Tikki	each of 85 gm.	106
Palak Puri	each of 45 gm.	112
Salads	100 gm.	140
Fruits (100 gm)		
Apple		59
Apricot		53
Banana		116
Cherries		64
Dates (dried)		317
Grapes (black)		58
Grapes (green)		70
Grape fruit		17

(Contd.)

(Contd.Table)

Fruits (100 gm)		
Musk Melon		16
Guava		51
Sweet lime		35
Mango ripe		34
Water Melon		16
Raisins		305
Orange (peeled)		48
Papaya (raw)		32
Peach		50
Pear / Plum		52
Pineapple		46
Pomegranate		65
Custard Apple		104
Juices		
Lemon juice (half lemon)	10 gm	6
Lemon juice with honey	250 ml	22
Honey water	10 gm (1 tsp)	32
Tender Coconut water	200 ml (one glass)	50
Carrot juice	250 ml(one glass)	120
Mausambi juice	-do-	160
Papaya juice	-do-	50
Grape juice	-do-	115
Orange juice	-do-	145
Pineapple juice	-do-	125

(Contd.)

(Contd. Table)

Juices		
Sugarcane juice	-do-	140
Fruit cocktail canned	120 gm	100
Tomato juice	One small glass	60
Custard apple juice	One small glass	70
Baked / Boiled vegetables	100 gm	50-80
Soups	250 ml	16-35
Mint Chutney	1 tsp	15-20
Hara Dhania	1 tsp	5-10
Raita	100 gm	50-80
Sprouts (Groundnut /Green gram)	50 gm	60-80
Leafy Vegetables (100 gm)		
Agathi		93
Bathua		30
Cabbage		27
Celery		37
Coriander		44
Curry leaves		108
Methi leaves		49
Lettuce		21
Mint		48
Parsley		87

(Contd.)

(Contd. Table)

Leafy Vegetables (100 gm)	
Radish leaves	28
Spinach	26
Carrot greens	77
Beet greens	46
Onion stalk	41
Roots and Tubers / Other Vegetable	
Beet root	43
Carrot	48
Potato	97
Onion	50
Radish	17
Sweet Potato	120
Turnip	29
Yam	110
Pumpkin	10
Tinda	21
Tomato green	23
French Beans	26
Brinjal/ Capsicum	24
Cauliflower	30
Cucumber	13
Lady's finger	35
Papaya green	27

(Contd..)

(Contd. Table)

Caloric Value of Milk and Milk Products		
Milk (buffalow)	One cup	210
Cow milk	One cup	130
Cow milk with 1 tsp honey	One cup	160
Milk shake	250 ml	210
Ghee	1 tsp	50
Butter	1 tsp	35
Butter milk	250 ml	40
Soya milk	250 ml	260
Sugar / Sweets / Spread / Oils/ Cakes-Pastries		
Sugar	1 tsp	20
Honey	2 tsp	30
Milk Chocolate	2 pc (40 gm)	210
Ice cream (vanilla /strawberry)	1 cup	160
Rassogulla (medium size)	One	120
Fruit cake	50 gm	175
Choco cake	50 gm	225
Custard	135 gm	375
Apple piece	85 gm (one)	260
Popcorn	1 Pack (250 gm)	148
Tea / Coffee with milk and sugar	One cup	50

(Contd.)

(Contd.Table)

Sugar / Sweets / Spread / Oils/ Cakes-Pastries		
Salt Biscuits	4	100
Cream crackers	3	100
Potato crisp	Pack of 35 gm	185
Soya / Groundnut Oil	1 tablespoon	40
Sunflower/Safflower Oil	1 tablespoon	43

Cereals(100gm)		*Protein (gm)*
Rice (Raw milled)		6.8
Wheat		11.8
Wheat flour (whole)		12.1
Wheat bread (white)		7.8
Wheat bread Brown)		8.8
Pulses –Bengal gram daal		20.8
Bengal gram roasted		22.5
Cowpea		24.0
Green gram		24.0
Red gram		22.5
Soya bean		42.0
Almond	100 gm	20.80
Cashew nut	100 gm	21.20
Ground nut	100 gm	24.5

9

Caloric Restriction Diet Plan

Conventional caloric-restriction diets induce low serotonin, its true. The excess insulin and low serotonin are a threat to good health. Good calories prevent both of these signals from developing. A caloric-restriction program is suggested if you need to lose less than 5 kilogram weight and have normal insulin. Remember, eating serotonin-stimulating foods will transform caloric restriction and turn it into easy to follow program because you no longer suffer from the food carvings, depression and irritability of low serotonin. You will lose weight faster than you would with conventional caloric restriction. The clinical study that proved the effectiveness of Good Calories has also shown that they increased the rate of weight loss. Make sure to be very careful about eating Good Calories, otherwise you may find your serotonin chemistry is thrown off and for losing a few kilos is just too high a price to pay for that.

When You Don't Lose Weight on the Free-Eating Plan

If you do not lose weight on the free-eating programme, you must question yourself if you are following the programme faithfully. The following are some of the most common ways that dieters deprive themselves of the benefits of the unrestricted programme:

1. Not eating a large breakfast of only low-protein; Good Calorie carbohydrates.
2. Eating too much animal protein.
3. Combining protein or saturated fats with starches.
4. Snacking on Bad Calories.
5. Skipping meals.
6. Eating too much saturated fat.
7. Eating too little unsaturated fat.
8. Eating too late at night.

If you have violated any of the rules, you should start the free-eating programme again. If you have not violated these rules and you are not losing weight, it means you should consider the caloric-restriction program. It will be totally different from your image of dieting. Even caloric - restriction is made easier by Good Calories.

How to Relieve Stress?

Stressed women excrete essential vitamins and minerals that may be retained if insulin levels remain under control. When insulin levels are out of control, stressed women are more susceptible to the food addiction. The simple act of dieting floods a woman's body with stress-producing hormones. Prolactin is a hormone released during mental or physical stress. After dieting, a woman's prolactin rises by more than 50% while a man's prolactin remains unchanged. Dieting creates stress in women and makes it nearly impossible for them to make enough serotonin to withstand that stress, and it creates conditions that can lead to food addiction. Dieting women have a special need to reduce stress in their lives. There are three techniques for lowering the stress: Exercise, Meditation and breathing. Reducing stress is a powerful tool to boost your physical and mental health, which makes weight-loss easier and helps to protect a woman's source of personal power.

Exercise

Most weight-loss programmes recommend exercise as a means to burn excess calories. Unfortunately, many of these programmes can be excessive for some women due to unbalanced plan disturbing the functioning of serotonin and insulin. However, you should not overdo exercise. Many dieting women attack their bodies with such a fury of exercise that prolactin, serotonin, and other important hormones go into the stress mode. All you need is a thirty minutes of exercise every day. You can do more, but only if you gradually build up to a higher level. *Remember, Over-exercising is Harmful.* This programme does not recommend high-intensity exercise. Instead, the following guidelines are suggested:

1. Find an exercise you enjoy.

2. Exercise for at least 30 minutes, five times per week.

3. Do not overdo it. Never exercise to exhaustion.

What Type of Exercise Should be Adopted?

Dieting women usually ask this question. Repetitive muscle movements are most effective at elevating serotonin. Walking, aerobic and running are highly recommended forms of exercise. Ancient *'Hatha Yoga'* and tai chi are also excellent forms of exercise for overweight persons. These ancient disciplines are based on a balanced approach to fitness, especially useful for the entire mind-body connection. These forms of exercise make you feel energized, calm and revitalized. The best form of exercise for an housewife to maintain her body is one that you must do: *walking, jogging, gardening, playing golf, dancing—do anything that gets you moving.*

Meditation

Meditation is the ultimate way to reduce stress. It has the following effects:

1. Lowering heart rate and blood pressure.

2. Reduces the hormones associated with stress, prolactin and glucocorticoids.

3. Counters a dieting woman's tendency toward depression and low serotonin.

4. Lowers the thyroid-stimulating hormones (TSH), which create depression.

5. Activity of the neurotransmitters that oppose serotonin.

What is Meditation and How To Do It Correctly?

The beginners often ask this question. Meditation is like concentration, something we already do all the time. Concentration is necessary to accomplish anything in life. When you do something, you are concentrating. If you don't

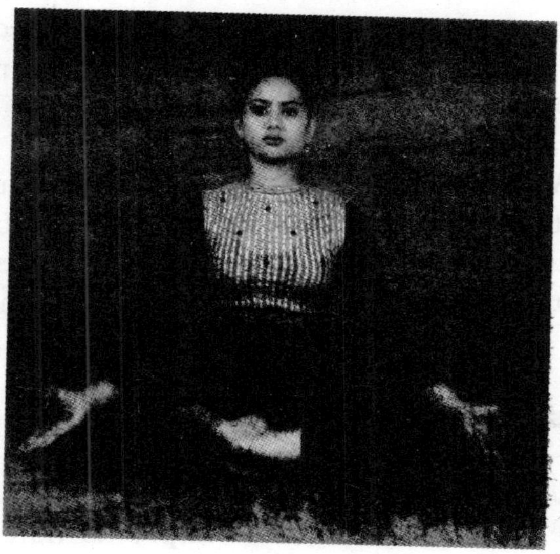

concentrate when you are driving, your vehicle will play havoc on the road. If you don't concentrate when reading, the words don't make sense. If you don't concentrate on your work, you are not productive. Concentration is the continued flow of our attention on an object or activity. You will like to know difference between concentration and meditation- which is the direction of focus. Whereas concentration is externally directed, meditation is directed to our innerself.

Breathing and Mantra

Proper breathing and a mantra are tools to help us experience meditation. It doesn't occur only while sitting in a certain posture. A meditative experience can happen anytime, anywhere. It can be done quietly and inconspicuously. Remember that meditation is simply the flow of our attention towards our inner self. Your inner self accompanies you everywhere, whether you are sitting in meditation, cooking meals in kitchen or negotiating in a boardroom.

A *'mantra'* is a phase to help you enter meditation more easily. The connection between meditation and mantra is strong. Simply repeating the mantra silently lets you immediately enter into a more meditative awareness.

What is 'Hamsa' Mantra?

Use of '*Hamsa*' mantra is very simple, also extremely powerful and as simple as listening to your breath. If you listen closely while you are breathing, you can hear its subtle sound — Hamsa. 'Ham' (pronounced hamm) is the sound incoming breath makes. Whereas 'Sa (pronounced saahh) is the sound of the outgoing breath. As you focus on the sound of the breath and listen to the sound of Hamsa, it might help you to know that *Hamsa is the actual vibrational sound of one's inner self.* As we listen to it, we remember and honor the truth within us. Observing your breath in this way leads to relaxation. When you change your breathing pattern you change your emotional state as described below:

- When you are angry you alternate between holding your breath and taking deep gulps of air.
- When you are nervous or afraid, your breath will be rapid and shallow.
- When you sit down to relax after exerting yourself, you take a long, deep breath.
- When you are calm, your breathing is even, deep and slow.

You breath mirrors your thoughts and emotions. If you don't want to use Hamsa mantra, you can simply focus on your breath, which can give you an enormous boost of energy and mental clarity. The way you breathe during meditation is the way you naturally breathe when you are calm: slowly, evenly and deeply. Breathing this way makes your mind receptive to meditation.

Correct Meditation Techniques

1. Breathe deeply.
2. Coordinate the mantra with the rhythm of your breathing.
3. As you inhale, silently repeat 'ham'.
4. As you exhale, silently repeat 'sa'.
5. Hear these sounds in your breath.
6. Now you are ready to start regular meditation sessions.

It helps to meditate at approximately the same time each day. Early mornings and late evenings before going to bed are excellent times because the environment is generally quieter. Whatever time you choose, try to be regular. It is helpful to sit at the same place every day. Ideally, you should meditate in a quiet room in which you can be alone. If you don't have that luxury just find a quiet corner and make it your meditative heaven. Begin with 15 minutes. Sit comfortably either on the floor with your legs crossed or in a chair maintaining a relaxed, comfortable, upright position. Your back and neck should be straight, without stiffening your muscles, to allow for full, deep breathing. Meditation will give you the ability to experience the calm that lies beyond the mind.

Advanced Exercises: Breath Retention

For those who already meditate and want a more advanced breathing technique, a new mediator should not attempt these until he/she feels comfortable with basic meditation.

Serotonin Chemistry and Diet

All conventional diets lower a woman's serotonin. High-protein, low-fat and high carbohydrate diets all bring on abnormal serotonin. Even conventional serotonin-boosting diets fail to meet women's need, and may lower serotonin. There are serotonin-stimulating drugs available in the market, but these carry the risk of many harmful and even fatal side effects. Women must eat foods that sustain their serotonin chemistry and restore its level to normal. There are two programmes that support a woman's serotonin, increase her well-being and allow her to lose weight.

1. *Serotonin and a woman's psyche*: Women need different foods because their brains have much more serotonin than men. Female brains have a greater storage capacity, thus generally more developed than in the male. This is because of female sex hormones, which enhance serotonin activity. The higher levels among women may cause importance for functions such as appetite, sexuality, cooperative attitude, impulsive behavior and aggression. Low serotonin creates a sense of panic, anxiety and depression in female sex. The symptoms of low serotonin include weight gain, depression, stress, tendency toward substance abuse, pre-mature sex, food cravings and eating disorders, sexual dysfunction, anxiety, irritability, disturbed

sleep, headaches, obsessive and compulsive behavior, inability to form proper social relationship and lower social dominance.

2. *Supporting a woman's serotonin*: Because women have more serotonin, they have a greater need to eat foods that support serotonin synthesis. Without these foods, their capacity to have slim, healthy bodies and potential power will decline. Low serotonin creates various problems in women such as increased appetite, pre-occupation with food, binge eating, depression, irritability, sleep disorders, impulsive behavior and eating disorders, such as anorexia and bulimia. Studies reveal, women who go on semi-starvation, weight-loss diets for few months have several problems with mood, lethargy, depression, irritability and decreased feelings of energy.

How to Control Low Serotonin?

Insulin controls serotonin synthesis. It causes stored tryptophan and amino acid to be released and transported into the brain where it is converted into serotonin. Insulin controls the blood sugar created by carbohydrates. Therefore, carbohydrates elevate serotonin. Chocolate, sweets, bread, sugars and starches are rich in carbohydrates.

10

Vitamins and Minerals For Your Body

What is a Vitamin?

Vitamin is not a food but is usually present in the foods we eat. Nor it is so-called 'food supplement'. If you eat nothing but vitamins, you would soon starve. Vitamins do not provide energy, nor do they build up worn out tissue. Still without vitamin you cannot live. Vitamins play a very important part in most chemical reactions within the body. Where do vitamins come from? First of all, they are built up in plants and they are found in all fresh foods. However, some vitamins especially vitamin C, can be destroyed by prolonged cooking. Drying or exposure to sun and wind, too, destroy its properties. Other vitamins are not so easily destroyed, and will stand cooking and boiling. Vitamins work in various ways, and are often closely related to each other in their reaction within the body. Most vitamins do not occur alone and are often found in pairs or groups.

Vitamin A : Vitamin A is the 'Beauty Vitamin'. It helps to keep the skin smooth and soft. It is also needed for the mucous membranes lining in the nose, throat and bronchial tubes as well as the entire digestive tract, the bladder, kidneys and pelvic organs. Vitamin A aids in the normal growth of bones and teeth, particularly in children and young people.

When Vitamin A is lacking, the skin becomes thick and rough, the eyes appear dull and lusterless. Infections arise in various parts of the body. Kidney and bladder stones are most common in people whose diets are deficient in vitamin A. The vitamin helps to fight infectious diseases. It keeps eyes bright and without adequate vitamin A our vision would soon be impaired. Vitamin A is formed from a chemical substance known as carotene, which is present in all green leafy vegetables, especially coriander and amaranth leaves, and also in fruits and vegetables such as carrot, squash, sweet potato, pumpkin, apricot, papaya, mango, avocado, melon and nearly all yellow fruits. Any diet containing an abundance of fresh fruits and vegetables will be rich in vitamin A.

Vitamin B Complex : It belongs to the family of vitamins B, which has more than a dozen of vitamins — all different and performing a wide variety of functions working together for the benefit of body. Because of close bond between them, they are eventually referred to as B complex vitamins. Cereals, such as rice, wheat and barley—all contain B complex vitamins. But they are particularly found in the outer covering of the grain. As such polished rice and white flour from wheat lose most of these important vitamins.

Vitamin B_1 (Thiamine) : They are one of the most important vitamins required by the body. It enters into almost every chemical reaction within the body. Without thiamine, the cells cannot utilize oxygen or fuel for energy. The nervous system cannot function properly without thiamine, nor can the muscles perform at their best. When thiamine is absent from the diet, muscle pains develop over the body. The nerves become irritable and the individual suffers from digestive disturbances, weakness, anemia and lack of appetite. The trouble is almost always due to poor diet.

The best sources of vitamin B_1 are whole-grain cereals such as bread, flour, breakfast foods, wheat germ, red rice, unpolished and parboiled rice, rice polishing, brewer's yeast, fresh fruits, eggs, vegetables, dried beans, peas and lentils. Thiamine is absent from most refined foods such as white flour, white sugar, starch, unpolished rice and fats. Vitamin B_1 cannot be stored in the body and must be included in the diet every day.

The use of soda in cooking destroys this vitamin and therefore should be avoided. Growing children, nursing mothers and women who are pregnant, all need extra amounts of vitamin B_1.

Vitamin B_2 (Riboflavin) : This type of vitamin enables the body to use carbohydrates. When riboflavin is absent from the diet, chronic sores develop at the angles of the mouth and may cause an abnormal shiny redness of the lips, burning in the eyes and discoloration of the tongue. Best sources of vitamin B_2 are milk, egg, beans, peas, pulses, yeast, whole-grain products and green leafy vegetables. This vitamin is easily lost when the food is cooked with too much water.

Niacin (Nicotinic Acid) : It is very important for the skin and also for the central nervous system. When niacin is absent, the serious condition known as pellagra develops. The skin becomes rough, and the patients suffer from a gradual loss of strength and have mental depression and so-called 'neurasthenia'. The skin becomes rough and scaly, and becomes dark. Other symptoms include soreness in the tongue, burning sensation in the mouth and throat. The patient complains of nervousness, dizziness, insomnia, muscular weakness and foul stools. Prevention is not difficult. Any well-balanced diet will be adequate in niacin. Foods, such as milk, eggs, fruits, groundnuts, fresh green vegetables and whole grains provide sufficient niacin to maintain good health.

Vitamin B_6 (Pyridoxine) : This vitamin is found in yeast, whole grains, rice polishing, bran, all legumes, pulses, egg yolk and milk. Lack of vitamins in the diet, young babies may develop convulsions. Adults suffer from extreme nervousness and irritability.

Vitamin B_{12} : It is very important in the production of red blood cells. The lack of vitamin causes anemia. The patient may feel pain, tingling and numbness in the extremities and there may be partial paralysis. A well-balanced diet, that include milk provides ample vitamin B_{12}

Vitamin C (Ascorbic Acid) : Vitamin C is the great healing vitamin of the body particularly needed by those suffering from severe infection and prolonged illness. When vitamin C is absent from the diet, a serious disease known as scurvy develops. The bones become painful and tender, and pinpoint hemorrhages develop under the skin. Scurvy is sometimes seen in pregnant women, nursing mothers and women who live on restricted diets. Vitamin C cannot be stored in human body, it must be taken every day. Best sources of vitamin C are orange, Indian gooseberries, lemon, lime, guava, tomato and potato.

Vitamin D : It is needed in the development of strong, healthy bones to maintain the right concentration of calcium and phosphorus within the body. This vitamin is particularly important in babies and young children, whose bones are developing rapidly. Vitamin D is often called the 'sunshine vitamin' because ultraviolet rays of the sun produce this vitamin. When vitamin D is absent from the diet, serious bone deformities occur. In children, this condition is known as rickets. The bones become soft and easily bent and the joints lose their shape. Premature babies are more prone to have rickets. The danger is great to dark-skinned children who live in cool climates. Rickets occur more frequently in winter months. Breast-fed babies are more likely to develop this disease, when mothers not on a well-balanced diet. Best sources of vitamin D are egg yolk, fish-liver oil and milk. Human body produces much of its own vitamin D.

Vitamin E : It has something to do with the reproductive functions of the body. Vitamin E is found in whole-grain cereals, green vegetables, olive oil, coconut oil and other vegetable oils. Doctors prescribe vitamin E for certain heart conditions. Any well-balanced diet contains sufficient vitamin E to meet normal needs of the body.

Vitamin K : It is essential in the clotting of the blood. When it is absent, prolonged bleeding may occur and severe anemia may result. Vitamin K is abundant in all green vegetables and also in soybeans and tomatoes. Hemorrhages may occur when this vitamin is missing from the diet. Some doctors prescribe vitamin K prior to surgery and advise its use during pregnancy to prevent severe hemorrhage after childbirth. All well-balanced diets contain vitamin K.

The Minerals and Your Body

The minerals in human body have many important functions to perform. Calcium and Phosphorus are needed for building strong bones and teeth. In the absence of both minerals, the body would quickly collapse. Many different minerals are found within the body, most of them in very small amounts, known as 'trace metals'. Some minerals like cobalt and copper are important minerals. But there are four minerals — calcium, phosphorus, iron and iodine — those are very important. We need much larger quantities of these and must be included in the diet for maintaining good health.

Calcium : Calcium or lime is the most abundant mineral in the body. Almost all the calcium is found in the bones, where it provides strength and stability to the whole system. A small quantity of calcium is always carried in the blood stream, where among other things, it helps to prevent serious hemorrhages. Calcium is also necessary for nerves and muscles. When the calcium level in the body drops below the safe level, the nerves become extremely irritable and the muscles go into spasm. Cramping pains may then be felt in various parts of the body, particular in the larger muscles of the legs. But nowhere is calcium more important than in the muscles of the heart. When calcium is reduced in the blood stream, the heart quickly loses its power, becomes irregular and may even stop beating altogether. Calcium is vital to health.

Young mothers need extra calcium, particularly during pregnancy and the nursing period. It is important for children and young people whose bones are growing rapidly. Calcium deficiency in the body causes diseases like 'rickets' in children and 'osteomalacia' in adults. Child's normal development is retarded due to weakness in the bones. Both rickets and osteomalcia can be cured by taking adequate quantity of calcium, phosphorus and vitamin D. Best sources of calcium are milk, dairy products, green vegetables, peas, beans, soybeans, eggs, lentils, potatoes and fish.

Phosphorus : Phosphorus is another essential mineral having much to do with the functions of all body cells. It is associated with other important substances, such as enzymes, proteins and carbohydrates. Phosphorus is necessary for muscles and helps to maintain the normal acid-base balance of the body. It is essential in building sound healthy teeth and bones. Phosphorus is found in all foods which are rich source of calcium. It is also present in whole-grain cereals, legumes and nuts, and is particularly abundant in milk (where it is associated with calcium) especially for children and the nursing mothers.

Iron : Iron is very important mineral for the body. Most of the iron is found in the red blood cells, where it forms part of that very complex protein known as hemoglobin. This is the red substance that gives color to the blood. It carries oxygen to the tissues and keeps us alive. Red blood cells are extremely small. Normally, there are around 5,000,000 cells in a drop of blood. Each red cell contains 250,000,000 molecules of hemoglobin and 1,000,000,000 atoms of iron. In few seconds during which, the tiny red cell is passing through the lung, it picks up 1,000,000,000 molecules of oxygen from the air. At the same time it drops 1,000,000,000 molecules of carbon dioxide brought in from the tissues of the body. Unwanted carbon dioxide is then removed from the body as we exhale or breathe out. So we keep breathing fresh air to supply the red cells with oxygen to replace the carbon dioxide. We call this respiration.

Most cells in the body live for years, perhaps even for life. However, red cells in the blood, soon wear out from the strain. Red cells last only about four months, and then are destroyed. They are replaced with new cells. Each tiny red cell carries its own little portion of iron. It is known fact that iron rusts when it is exposed to the air. Rusting is even more rapid when the air is damp. This chemical reaction is known as oxidation. A molecule of iron attaches itself to a molecule of oxygen from the air, forming iron oxide. This is exactly what happens when the red blood cells pass through lungs. The air within lungs is warm and damp, and the iron in the red cells rusts as it passes through lungs. From there the cells are carried by the blood stream to the heart and pumped to all the parts of the body. In fact, iron is very important to the well being of all parts of the body.Green leaves, egg, apricot, raisins, potatoes, oatmeal, whole-grain, cereals and liver are all good source of iron.

Iodine : Like other minerals, iodine is found in the foods we eat. From the digestive tract, the iodine passes into the blood stream and is soon picked up by the thyroid. Common table salt, known as sodium chloride is highly important in maintaining the normal acid base balance of the body. If a person has kidney or heart trouble, his salt intake may have to be somewhat restricted, especially if he has high blood pressure. Oedema or swelling of legs and ankles may occur when there is too much salt in the body.

11

Total Body Care by Diet and Nutrition

Precautions When Cooking Food

Cooking is an art as well as a science. Properly cooked food should be clean, hygienic and free from contaminants. Preserve all nutrients such as vitamins, minerals and other vital organic substances. Cooking of food primarily improves its taste, flavor, makes it easily digestible and destroy the micro-organism present. For retaining nutritive value of the food the following simple rules are followed:

1. Wash vegetables thoroughly before cutting.

2. Cut vegetables just before cooking.

3. Use sufficient water for cooking.

4. Serve cooked food immediately after preparing.

5. Vegetable salad should be prepared just before serving to save vitamin C.

6. Fruits and vegetables should be eaten as far as possible in their natural form.

7. Soup could be prepared from the leftover water after boiling the vegetable.

8. Use stainless steel vessels for cooking food.

Nutritive Value of Food

There is sufficient effect on nutritive value of food when cooking. The vitamins and minerals loose 10 to 60% nutritive value as a result of improper cooking.

1. *Carbohydrate*: Cooking helps in proper digestion of starch, which when cooked smells up and gets gelatinized and is digested in the body easily.

2. *Fat*: Ordinary cooking have little effect on fat, whereas deep frying may lead to destruction of essential fatty acid and formation of toxic substances.

3. *Proteins*: Application of moderate heat splits protein and shrinks it to make it easily

digestible. But severe heat such as roasting, baking and frying reduces its nutritive value.

4. *Vitamins*: Vitamin A and D has very little destruction during cooking due to oxidation by air. However, frying and roasting cause considerable loss. Loss in vitamin C occurs by oxidation due to exposure to air. The quantity of vitamin C lost during cooking varies from 10 to 60% depending upon the vegetable cooked and method of cooking.

5. *Minerals*: Loss in minerals (Calcium, Iron and Phosphorus) occurs when excess cooking water is discarded. Loss of nutritive iron contents during cooking occurs. When vegetables are cut with iron knives, appreciable amount of iron incorporates on vegetable. Similarly, iron percentage increases by roasting on hot iron pans.

Effect Due to Different Methods of Cooking

The following effects on the nutrients present in foods, due to different methods of cooking have been registered:

1. Cooking by water causes loss of vitamin C. If excess water is used, 30 to 70% water-soluble vitamins and minerals are lost.

2. Cooking by steam causes slight loss of vitamin C and negligible losses of other vitamins.

3. Cooking in pressure cooker results in moderate loss of vitamin C and slight loss of vitamin B 12)

4. Deep fat frying results in destruction of Thiamin, vitamin A carotene and vitamin C.

5. Shallow frying causes moderate loss of vitamin C and slight loss of vitamin A carotene and thiamin.

6. Dry roasting leads to heavy loss of thiamin and reduces nutritive value of protein. However, roasting of groundnut causes slight loss in nutritive value of protein.

7. Cooking soda added to food causes severe loss of Thiamin (about 70%)and Riboflavin (about 30%).

8. Sprouting of pulses increase the vitamin C content and also the digestibility of pulse.

Cooking has several advantages. It improves the food palatability, quality and digestibility. Following precautionary measures could minimize the loss of vitamins and minerals when cooking:

Vegetarianism Vs Non-vegetarianism

Non-vegetarian food is still considered most important in daily diet. The only good thing about non-vegetarian food is the presence of complete protein, which causes heavy work to the kidneys, which in turn lessens the efficiency of the organs leading to degenerative disorders.

1. Death rate among non-vegetarians by coronary heart disease has been recorded higher as compared to the vegetarian because of higher levels of cholesterol and fat absorbed into the system through non-vegetarian diet.

2. Non-vegetarian food adds calories and lead to obesity, diabetes and high blood pressure.

3. The tissues of all animals contain poisonous wastes. Hence when the non-vegetable food is consumed, toxic level in the system increases. Remember, soyabean is a better substitute to meat.

4. Non-vegetarian food items kept in cold storage and reheated result in rapid decomposition since the non-vegetarian diet is relatively low in fiber content.

5. The movement of food in bowels slows down resulting in exposure to the large intestine

to toxins present in the non-vegetarian food leading to risk of colon cancer.

6. A well-selected vegetable diet can supply good quality protein if the following method isfollowed and such food definitely be superior to the non-vegetable diet. Combine legumes (dried peas, beans, peanuts etc) with grains (barley, wheat, rice etc).

Nutrition Value of Foods We Eat

1. *Coffee*: A cup of coffee early in the morning (particularly in winter) boost up one's spirit. This is because the caffeine present in the coffee stimulates the adrenal gland to release. Adrenaline into blood stream raises the blood pressure, blood sugar and increases the pulse and heart rates. A single cup of coffee contains up to 100 mg of caffeine. Most common problems faced by coffee consumers are insomnia, slightly raised blood pressure and inability to relax.

2. *Tea*: Contains toxin (a toxic chemical which contains caffeine to some extent).

3. *Colas and Chocolates*: These, too, contain caffeine to some extent and have to be strictly avoided during dieting period. They cause health problems and also interfere

16.2. *Amla*: This miracle fruit immensely rich in pectin is the richest source of Vitamin C. It is cooling, diuretic and laxative in nature.

3. *Banana*: It contains appreciable amount of vitamin (A,B,C and D), calcium, magnesium, phosphorus, iron and copper.

4. *Figs*: Contains high sugar content. It relieves constipation.

5. *Grapes*: A revitalizing fruit, which contains ample protein, carbohydrates, vitamin A and B and minerals. It helps in elimination of toxins from the system and purify blood as well as increase the alkalinity of blood.

6. *Grape fruit*: It is largest of the citrus variety fruit available (source of potassium, vitamin A and vitamin B).

7. *Guava*: Very rich in vitamin C and regulates bowel movement.

8. *Lemon*: A citrus fruit rich in citric acid and alkaline. After complete digestion vitamin C in the lime juice strengthens connective tissues of the joints, improves the vitality and is very useful in treating cold, running nose and cough.

9. *Mango*: Rich in vitamin A and C. It cures diabetes and obesity.
10. *Water melon*: Being low in calories, it is ideal for weight watchers. Its cooling, refreshing and rich in vitamin C.
11. *Muskmelon*: Rich in alkaline salt. Treats hyperacidity, ulcers and other digestive disorders.
12. *Orange*: Rich in vitamin A, B and C and calcium. It is digestive and excellent blood purifier.
13. *Papaya*: Highly alkaline and digestive. Rich in vitamin A, B, C and D.
14. *Pomegranate*: Rich in sugar, iron and citric acid. Relieves constipation and prevent diarrhea.
15. *Pineapple*: Helps in digestion. Pineapple juice contains substance, almost similar to pepsin present in stomach. It raises alkaline and purify blood.
16. *Pear*: Contains more sugar and less acid. It is useful in case of bladder stone.
17. *Sapota (Cheeku)*: A high calorie fruit; hence diabetics and those having obesity should avoid. It is useful in relining constipation.

18. *Custard apple*: A high calorie sweet fruit; hence should be avoided by diabetics and obese patients.

19. *Dry fruits:* When soaked in water they retain their original fresh fruit forms.

20. *Vegetables*: These are consumed in the form of leaf, stem, root and flower. They are either used raw or after cooking. Root and tuber vegetables are rich in carbohydrates, low in fat and protein. Important root and tuber vegetables are beetroot, carrot, potato, sweet potato, radish, turnip, onion, garlic, ginger etc.

    Beetroot are juicy and rich in alkaline salts. It is good source of potassium, sodium, magnesium and iron. Radish is a very low calorie vegetable and has diuretic effect. Turnip is a rich source of calcium. Carrot is rich in vitamin A and gives a good color to the skin, helps in case of anemia, is a good blood purifier. Carrot juice is very useful for asthmatics, hyperacidity patients, under nourished people and treating ulcer. Potato contains starch, and alkaline consisting of approx. 70% moisture, 20% carbohydrates, 2% protein and minerals such as potassium and magnesium. It is a good source of vitamin C.

    Onion is classified under spice category, has a medical value also. It reduces cholesterol levels and is also a powerful antiseptic. Garlic has remarkable curative properties, which help to bring down cholesterol and release flatulence gas from the stomach. Ginger contains 80% moisture, little amount of protein and fiber. It is also carminative, stimulant, blood purifier and stimulate appetite.

Dietary Guidelines

- Excessive use of fruits and raw vegetables such as carrots, radish, lettuce, spinach, cauliflower, cabbage etc.

- Use of whole wheat such as brown bread, chapatis etc.

- Use of plenty of fibrous food such as beans, bran, leafy vegetables, oak flakes, china grass, Isabel etc.

- Generous intake of liquid such as water, lemon juice, fruit juices etc.

- Use of confectioneries, pastries, cakes, sweets etc should be curtailed.

- All dry fruits, figs, prunes and raisins. Use of apricot and plums, fresh fruits, banana, mango, grapefruit and orange should be encouraged.

- Taking 6 to 8 glasses of water immediately after getting up from bed stimulate bowel movement.

- Soaking dry fruits such as raisins, dates in the milk or plain water and taking it before going to bed at night or in the morning is very useful in the treatment of constipation.

- Mix 2-3 tsp of 'Isabgol' with milk or warm water either at bedtime or early in the morning is very useful.

12

Burn Fat Without Tears

Are You Overweight?

There are five categories of weight: Underweight, Healthy, Overweight, Obese and Very Obese. If you think you are overweight — but by how much? Refer the chart given in this book recommending the weight for men and women based on your height. You should weigh yourself on a reliable set of scales. Wear indoor clothing but not shoes. Maybe you're within the healthy weight range for your height but still feel flabby. In that case it's down to muscle tone and condition and it is very straightforward to get trim on exercise. But if you find yourself overweight then it is time to do something about it. A few simple changes in your lifestyle now could create a whole new sense of well-being and the figure to go with it. First though, we look at the reasons for the extra weight you are carrying.

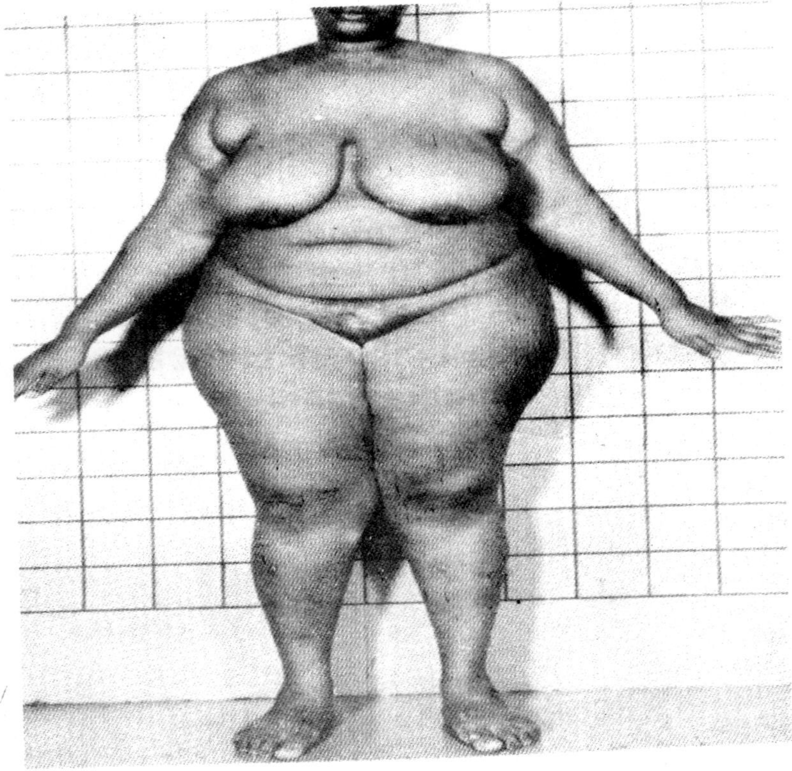

How Do You Become Overweight?

There is still lot to be learnt about obesity because even the experts disagree. It is possible that you are overweight because of genetic or hormonal reasons, in which case you should consult a doctor. Some experts believe that fat people have relatively slow metabolism — that their bodies burn energy at a much lower rate than leaner people of the same weight. Other experts suggest that overeating is the real problem, while another group claims that lack of exercise is to blame.

Let's Examine Some Facts

Most of the energy we get from food is used as fuel for normal body's functions and physical activities. This energy is measured in kilocalories, usually known as calories. The amount of energy we each require varies from person to person. For example, a construction worker might require 3500 calories a day, whereas a typist would need less than 2000. A substantial proportion, roughly about two-third of these calories are used to keep the body functioning and properly maintained. They provide energy for the vital organs such as heart, lungs, brain, liver and kidneys for digestion, for maintaining body temperature and for growth. The amount of energy expended in this way to keep the body well maintained is known as the Basal Metabolic Rate (BMR). The remaining calories provide energy for the physical activity, whether it is manual labor, housework or sports.

Some people burn energy more quickly than others; they have a higher BMR and this is closely linked to an individual. We become overweight when we eat more food than we need to maintain our BMR and fuel our physical activities. The excess energy intake is mainly stored as fat, a kind of reserve fuel tank in case of future food shortage. Generally, for most of us the shortage never arrives and unluckily, the excess fat builds up. There are people, who seem to eat huge amounts of food and stay slim. Studies reveal, some individuals burn more calories than others of equal weight, even when performing the same physical tasks and taking the same amount of rest. The hearty eaters, with higher BMR are seen much leaner than the people with lower BMR. Unfortunately, a slimming diet slows down the BMR. The digestion process itself requires 10% of the calories consumed and a very low calorie diet can produce a 15% drop in BMR. The body responds to starvation by slowing vital processes, so the less you eat, the less work your body does by itself. That is why it is important to exercise as well, and why a gradual reduction in calories is better than a starvation regime.

For many people, the weight problem starts in childhood. The guilt about being overweight can only be eased by the consolation of eating. The thought of being fat and unattractive often drives some people to indulge even more, because eating becomes the only pleasure left for them. Many nutritionists suggest that convenience foods are much to blame. Processed foods often lack nourishment.

Exercise— Is It Worth the Effort?

For some of us, even the thought of taking exercise is too much to bear. However, taking exercise does not have to be the same as doing exercises. We have seen that every kind of physical activity throughout the day requires energy – from walking downstairs to doing household work, even to making love. And the more energy you can use up, the less there will be left over to store as fat. The trouble is, that with today's lifestyle, it is really easy to avoid a great deal of activity. Automation and labor saving devices now replace much of the physical effort that would have been required in days gone by. This partly explains why levels of obesity and heart diseases have increased drastically in recent generation.

Do I Really Have To Exercise?

For a start, the sudden, extra demands on your body could be dangerous, especially if you are substantially overweight. The important is to find a type of exercise that you can happily maintain as part of your life, not just a get-slim-quick type of punishment that you will really hate after sometime. Perhaps you can think back to a sport or activity that you once enjoyed. Swimming, cycling and playing tennis or badminton is the excellent forms of exercise. Just 20 to 30 minutes or so, two or three times a week, is enough to get your system going and help to shed those extra kilos. Unfortunately, in today's fast life, majority of people can all make time to watch a regular TV programme or go to the pub to have sips, but no time to play sports or exercise.

If you really can't manage an hour or two for sport on a regular basis, then do think carefully about doing some simple exercises at home. Start with few simple exercises like Sit-ups, Waist stretches, stair hops and leg stretches in the beginning and gradually build-up to a worthwhile level of 15 or more a day. Once you have developed a reasonable degree of fitness.

What Else Can I Try to Get Slim?

The simplest way to start boosting your daily activity is to increase the amount of time you spend walking. But don't stroll, walk briskly, striding out, arm swinging. If you drive into town, park the car away from the center and walk the rest of the way. If you go by bus, get off at an earlier stop and walk up to the destination. There are so many little ways in which you can effectively increase your daily activity. You could spread some of your shopping throughout the week so that you walk to the local store each day. If you work in a office, take the stairs to the upper floor instead of the lift. Climb two stairs at a time — it's really a good exercise. Try and escape at lunch hours at the work place and walk round the market or a local park in the area. Remember, every bit of extra activity burns energy and boosts your BMR, so provided you are eating more than you need. The extra energy will eventually come from your reserves of fat.

By exercising regularly you will become physically fitter and although you will use up more energy you will find that it is replaced more quickly so that you actually feel more energetic and less tired. Indeed, exercise has a balancing effect on stress and anxiety. It is difficult to stay anxious or angry while your mind and body are occupied with physical activity. When doing vigorous exercise, powerful chemicals called to endorphins are released by brain. These act on the body in a similar way to morphine in producing a mental state. People who do regular exercise usually sleep more soundly, experience less aches and pains, feel generally calmer and have smaller appetites than inactive people. So with the right attitude to diet and exercise you really can set yourself on a slimmer, healthier and happier course for life.

Is it never too late ot start exercising?

But if you are seriously overweight, have suffered recent illness, have joint problems or have reached 40 or above, check with your doctor before you begin. Here are few exercise cautions:

1. Do start exercising slowly and build up gradually.

2. Don't push yourself to exhaustion. You should make yourself breathless but not speechless.

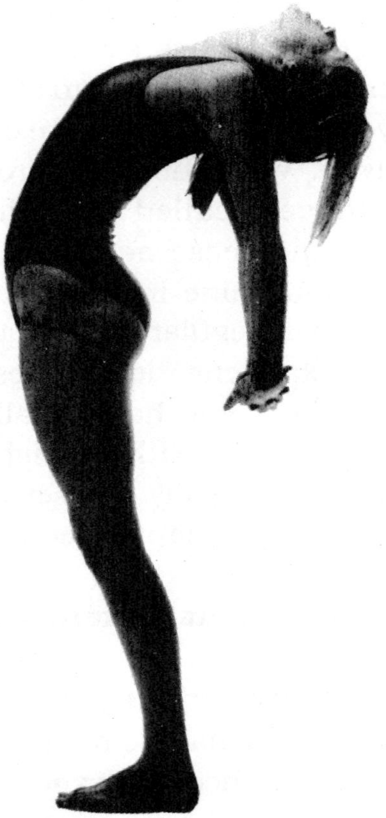

3. Do warm up and gently stretch before exercising.

4. Don't stop suddenly. Slow the pace to a comfortable level towards the end of the session.

5. Don't exercise after eating a meal, wait at least an hour before starting.

6. Don't ignore pain-your body is telling you to stop.

Ten Points to Feel Great – Look Good

1. Avoid saturated fat and keep intake of all fat to a minimum.

2. Avoid refined sugar whenever possible.

3. Keep up a healthy intake of dietary fibere.

4. Use fresh, unprocessed, ingredients as much as you can.

5. Try to keep to three meals a day. Stop thinking about eating.

6. Eat moderate portions. Try to eat slowly and chew thoroughly. Avoid over-eating, but at the same time don't starve yourself.

7. Maintain the recommended level of exercise and arrange your day to include plenty of activity – not just exercise.

8. Drink plenty of water and fruit juice. It does help to keep your appetite under control and 'flush out' bodily wastes and toxins.

9. Take time to enjoy your meal sitting at the table. Don't rush around or watch TV while eating. Try new recipes, taste exotic fruit and vegetables.

10. Celebrate your better shape with new clothes or an evening out. Once you do get started, it is surprising how much easier it becomes day by day to adopt the healthier habits that promise a slimmer figure and much greater vitality.

A Holistic Approach is Key to Overcome Overweight

If you have a health problem, and you treat only the symptom and not the underlying cause, you may experience temporary relief. But the symptom will likely return...again...and again. Sound anything like your extra kilos? The kilos you have lost and regained...again...and again? According to a renowned acupuncturist, overweight is the symptom of fundamental imbalances in your body, emotions and mind. These imbalances include:

1. *Emotional Imbalance*: in which food is used as a substitute for love or a way to 'stuff' your uncomfortable feelings back inside you.

2. *Nutritional Imbalance*: with the body crying out for the nutrients it needs for optimal functioning-nutrients that your food choices are not supplying.

3. *Physical Imbalance*: such as stored toxins in the digestive tract that drain your energy and cause you to eat 'stimulating' foods like sugar that makes you even more toxic in the long run.

4. *Mental Imbalance*: in which your thoughts anxiously or angrily or sadly dwell on the past or future and you are never mindful of what you are eating.

When you are in balance, you naturally and easily make food choices that support your overall state of health. Here are some of the tested methods for correcting the imbalances that are the underlying cause of overweight:

Food – that stops cravings: Light, smoothie or blender drink for breakfast is the most important balance-restoring step for many weight-loss people. The drink is a total infusion of essential vitamins, minerals, fatty acids, protein and fiber. And it is a great way to cut down on food cravings, because with the super-nutrition in the smoothie, you are giving your body the nutrients it needs. Your food cravings, as well as depression, irritability, anxiety and many other emotional and mental problems are the signs that your brain does not have enough of them. Just put the following ingredients in a blender, mix and drink:

Rice milk	1 cup
Soy milk	1 cup
Apple juice	1 cup
Orange or other fruit juice	1 cup
Banana and fresh strawberries	One and Four respectively
Blackstrap molasses	1 teaspoon
Aloe juice	1 tablespoon
Black cherry juice concentrate	1 tablespoon
Powdered green formulations	1 tablespoon
Powdered brewer's or nutritional yeast	1to2 tablespoon
Raw organic bee pollen (loose)	1 teaspoon
Flaxseed oil	1 tablespoon

Affirmations- that makes the right food choices : Making the right, healthy balanced choice is what your mind is thinking at that moment. Spend 5 to 10 minutes once or twice a day mentally affirming your intention to be balanced and healed. It is much more likely that you will make the right food choices. Choose one or two affirmations from the following:

- Reveal a clear, healthier, happier in you.
- Thinking control in yourself.
- Taking responsibility of your physical self, wellness and your health.
- Eat to nourish your mind, body and spirit.

Rebounding- the best weight-loss exercise: Jumping on a re-bounder or small trampoline is a particularly good exercise for those trying to lose weight. It helps strengthen the lymphatic system- the body system drains toxins and supports stronger immunity. Have an exercising session of 10 to 20 minutes of re-bounding three to five times a week.

Glutamine- balance blood sugar, stop cravings: Food cravings, particularly for sweets and starches, are often caused by low blood sugar or hypoglycemia. You can stabilize the delivery of blood sugar to your brain and stop the cravings or get relief of carbohydrate cravings with the help of medicines in consultation with your doctor.

Tyrosine- for low energy and poor concentration: When you feel fatigued and brain-fogged nearly all the time and use coffee, cigarettes and sweets to give you a lift. Experts usually recommend 500 to 2000 mg (start with 500 mg) of tyrosine three times day – before breakfast, at mid morning and at mid-afternoon (with the consultation of doctor) and you will feel energized and alert.

D-phenylalanine- if you eat to overcome emotional pain: Amino acid d-phenylalanine builds up your brain's reservoir of endorphins, the natural opiates that help to create feelings of pleasure and reduce physical pain. Plenty of high-protein foods are recommended which supply amino acids that manufacture endorphins.

GABA- for stress and tension: When the muscles are chronically tense, and you feel stressed and burned out, you need relaxation and calmness. If this sounds like this, you may need gamma amino-butyric acid (GABA). Don't take the supplement first thing in the morning, since it may make you too relaxed. Seek the guidance of your doctor. GABA taken in combination with glycine can be even more calming than GABA alone.

. **5-HTP- For Depression, Anxiety or Low Self-esteem**

If you have low levels of the brain chemical serotonin, you can have a host of emotional and mental problems that compel you to overeat sweets, starches and chocolate. This problem includes depression, anxiety, low self-esteem, obsessive thoughts, winter blues, irritability and insomnia. If you are experiencing any of above, you may take 50 to 100 mg of the serotonin - boosting supplement 5-hydroxy-tryptophan (5-HTP) three times a day in consultation with your doctor.

Fats That Can Help You Lose Weight Up to 20% Of Their Fat in Couple of Months

A deficiency of certain types of good fats, called essential fatty acids (EFA) that body requires can lead you to crave and overeat fats that put on extra weight. In fact 'Fat phobia' is the cause of so much overweight in our country. Remember, saturated fats in animal products and trans-fats in the processed foods like fatty fish, certain oils, leafy greens, avocados and nuts and seeds - all leave a harmful effect on body. The different types of EFA stimulate fat metabolism so that body burns excessive fat, trigger the production of hormones so that makes you feel full and balance your body's level of insulin (the hormone that burns sugars) so you don't crave high-calorie sugars and other fattening products carbohydrates. Here's what expert dieticians recommend:

FLAXSEED OIL: reset your thermostat: Alpha-linolenic acid (LNA) and other fatty acids found in flaxseed oil help reset your body's thermostat to a normal level, so you burn excess calories. They also help normalize insulin metabolism, thus reducing sugar cravings. 1 tablespoon a day with a meal is the recommended dose.

GLA: activate brown fat: Gamma-linolenic acid (GLA) helps you lose weight by activating dormant brown fat that helps burn excess calories. Brown fat makes it possible to expend ingested fat as energy rather than storing it as excess white fat. Fantastically successful results have been obtained due to this.

CLA: inhibit the enzyme that stores fat: The essential fatty acid conjugated linolenic Acid

(CLA) may help in your weight loss efforts. According to experts, people who take 3000 milligrams of CLA daily are seen lost about 20% of their body fat in three months without dieting. CLA has proved very effective in fighting breast cancer in females.

FISH OIL: to balance your overall fat intake: A medical study reveals that fatty acids available in fish oil are unable to reduce weight directly, but these help in balancing your overall intake of fats and maintain good health. The prescribed dosage is approximately 1000 milligrams two to three times a day preferably in consultation with a dietician.

Don't Skip Meals for Burning Fat

Fasting is used to cleanse the body of all the imbedded waste matter, remove the deep - rooted toxins and give rest to the different organs of the body. In order to prepare the body for fasting begin with eating only raw vegetables or fruits. Do not take more than four to five glasses of liquid diet a day. You are now ready for complete fasting. Take only fresh lime with honey or plain water. Never begin fasting suddenly nor end it suddenly. For the next four to five days take only raw or boiled vegetables. Over a period of ten days you can come back to your original cereal diet. Many of the ailments such as acme and pimples, rheumatism, asthma, ulcers, alcoholism, heart disease and many more disorders dissolve itself while fasting.

Eating too little will not make you thin. Ignore all the fat and very low-calorie diets. Don't skip meals – the optimum diet plan is five regular, small meals a day. If you want to eat more, eat in intervals and keep dinner as a light snack. Eat low fat and high fiber foods. Try to eat food, which derive no more than 20% of their calories from fat. One grain of fat equals nine calories.

Healthy Eating Pyramid

You will need to follow 'healthy eating pyramid' guidelines. If a food has 100 calories with four grams of fat, that means 36 calories from fat – almost 40%. Healthy eating pyramid recommends that between 35 and 40% of your diet should come from whole grains like cereals and brown bread, rice and pasta. Vegetables should form 15 to 25% of your daily intake, followed by fruits about 10 to 15%, then dairy products and meats, which should be only about 10% each. Added fats, oils and sweets should be no more than 5%.

The Optimum Diet Plan: Five Small Meals a Day

Follow these points carefully:

1. 'I do not eat' is incorrect diet plan. However, overeating is a cumulative process and

weight gain is the result. What you eat in a day or even a week won't make much difference, but over a year you will misjudge your food intake. An extra slice of bread a day over a year or two can make the difference between a lean body and a fat one.

2. Remember, a good food makes you thinner. The type of food you eat is as important as the amount. The biggest problem with traditional weight-loss diets is nutritional deficiency, which undermines your immune system, promotes diseases and if your diet lacks adequate vitamin and minerals, your body will want to eat more to make up for the deficiency. Varied diet regulates appetite.

3. You will like to know why diets make us fat. Every person has a body having own set point, a weight at which our body happily settles. Put weight on and it responds by burning energy faster. Lose weight and it burns calories more slowly in an effort to hang on to the set point.

4. Slow weight loss is best. Reduce your daily calorie level only a little, no more than 20% - just 400 calories off a 2000 a day diet. It means to lose around ½ kg to 1 kg a week

when you start that reduction to cut those calories from fat. When switching from low calorie to low fat diets, you do need to keep an eye on calories in general. The problem with low-fat diets is that people are tempted to eat unlimited low-fat diets.

Ten Essential Supplements to Fat Burning

These include:

1. Eat healthy diet.

2. Regular exercise.

3. Amino acids and enzymes crucial to fat-metabolism have found taking these as supplements may help you burn fat more efficiently.

4. Co-enzyme Q-10, a powerful nutrient is linked to the well being of every cell in the body. Q-10 aids energy production and possess fat burning properties. When the cells work at their optimum fat, is used as energy instead of being stored. 30 to 60 mg is recommended dosage.

5. Chromium Picolinate: This amino acid regulates insulin, the hormone that balances blood sugar levels. Those deficient in chromium may feel dizzy when hungry. 200 mg per day is recommended dosage.

6. Hydroxi-itric Acid (HCA): It encourages the production of glycogen from carbohydrates, which accumulates in the liver and muscles. It reduces appetite and increases energy levels in the body. HCA combined with an additional supplement like chromium can help the body burn existing fat to produce energy.

7. Green Tea: The body has two types of fat: Brown and Yellow. Yellow fat is visible below the surface of the skin whereas Brown fat sits against the skeleton in the upper part of body, and is metabolically active and triggers the metabolism of stored yellow fat. The yellow fat is responsible to increased calorie intake or to produce heat when the vital organs it. Constituents in green tea, readily available from health food shops, contribute to it. One to three cups of green tea per day is the recommended dosage.
8. L-Carnitine: An amino acid manufactured in the liver, has a vital role in helping the body transform fat into fuel. L-Carnitine's properties are greatly enhanced when taken before exercise. 500 to 1000 mg. per day is recommended dosage.

9. Lipotropic Factors: Nutrients which function in the liver as fat, prevent excessive build up of fat. Lipotropic factors are an aid to weight loss and help to reduce body fat and localized fat like cellulite.

10. Omega-3: These essential fatty acids reverse the weight gain, high cholesterol levels and risk of heart disease caused by saturated fats. Food rich in Omega-3 include fish oils, soybeans, linseeds and walnuts which help to reduce cholesterol and triglyceride levels, which should improve fat metabolism and aid weight loss. Vegetarians can take linseed oil instead of fish oil. 400 to 800 mg per day is the recommended dosage.

Sweating - The Fast Way to Burn Fat

You should aim to have three workouts a week, each consuming at least 300 calories. This is the estimated calorie-burning threshold at which you start to move body fat to make your pulse race and body sweat, and leave you feeling tired but exhilarated. Muscle is a fat-burning furnace taking centimeters off your waistline. Low-intensity exercise is just as effective, but you will need to work out for longer in order to get results.

Choose a fat-burning workout of your choice from different fat burning regimes. Strenuous swimming burns four times more calories than strenuous running. 20 minutes on the stair climber followed by 20 minutes of sit-ups develops a high-intensity regime that tone and firm chest, shoulders, back, arms, legs and feet. You can get enough oxygen to metabolize body fat and muscle. If you join a gym, choose one that is within walking distance of your home or workplace. A gym or health club is the perfect environment for exercising without distractions. Use the exercise bike, treadmill and rowing machine. Repetitive using light weights leads to increased muscle tissue. A recent study showed that or every two kg. muscle you build, you burn an extra 30 to 50 calories a day. Skating provides a better aerobic workout than cycling. You burn an average 285 calories during a 30- minute period of skating. A good exercise program will take into account not only the demands of your lifestyle but also of your body.

13

Burn Fat with Exercise and Low Calories Diets

An active lifestyle is the key to maintaining a youthful look, clear skin, supple body and vitality. Those who lead a sedentary lifestyle look and feel older more quickly than those who stay active, If you want to stay young, you can – but you have to work at it. There are people in their late 50's who look as good as if they were in their late 30's. Women who should be at the prime youth in 30's but sometimes look like they are in 50'. We can no longer dismiss this as merely the luck of genetics or the result of a pampered lifestyle. Once-taut tissue must inevitably sag, the skin will crinkle and loosen itself from its once-firm mooring. Although a decrease in taut in your skin is, to a certain extent, predetermined by your genetic make-up, it is possible to take timely steps to postpone the inevitable. If you want to stay young, stretch your way to a flexible, slim and trim body.

Chisel Away the Extra Flab

With this body-friendly sculpt and tone workout that boosts endurance, increases flexibility, and shapes you from fat to firm to fit. At the same time, leave enough time for the muscles to rest and recuperate, and optimize your physical and mental health.

Warm-up Exercises

Perform low-impact aerobic moves for 5 to 10 minutes before beginning the workout. Take a quick walk around your residential place or place of doing warm-up exercises or dance to your favorite tunes. The aim is to raise your core body temperature. After the warm-up, stretch the body muscles and move into the exercise routine. Here are few easy to do warm-up exercises:

Chair Pose / Utkata Posture (High, Mighty or Superior)

Stand straight. Keep feet and knees together. Bend knees as you lower your body down until thighs are parallel to the floor and imagine you are sitting on a chair. Now stretch your arms upwards joining palms. Hold for 10 minutes. Repeat exercise for 3-4 times. This exercise strengthens the ankles, calves, arms, legs, inner thighs and back.

Tree Pose (Vriksha Asana)

Stand straight with weight distributed evenly over both feet. Stretch arms up. Place right foot on your left upper thigh. Once you have attained balance, place your palms together in prayer position, at your chest or raise them over the

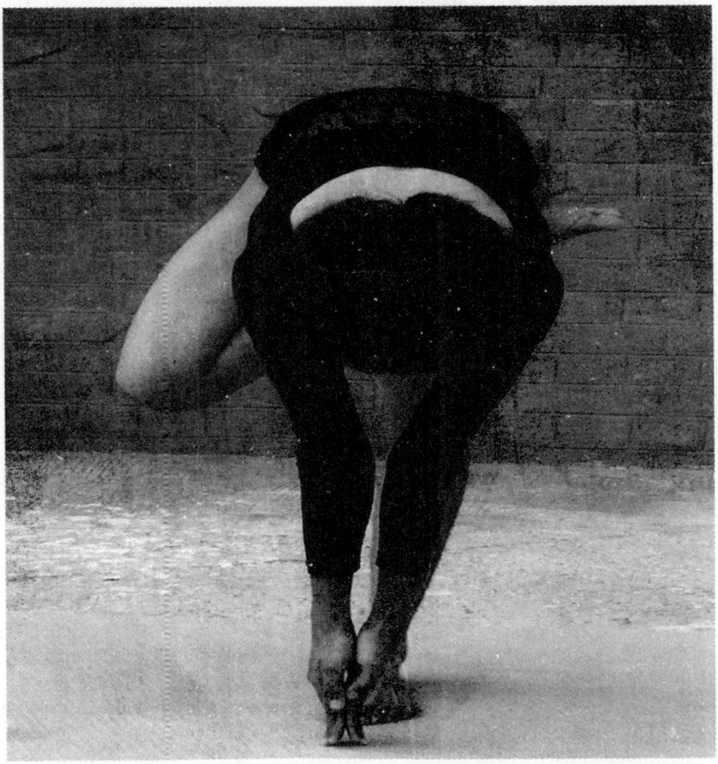

(Position-1)

head. Take a few deep-breath. Lower your right leg and repeat the exercise on the other side. This exercise corrects posture, improves concentration and balance, strengthen legs, arms and shoulders

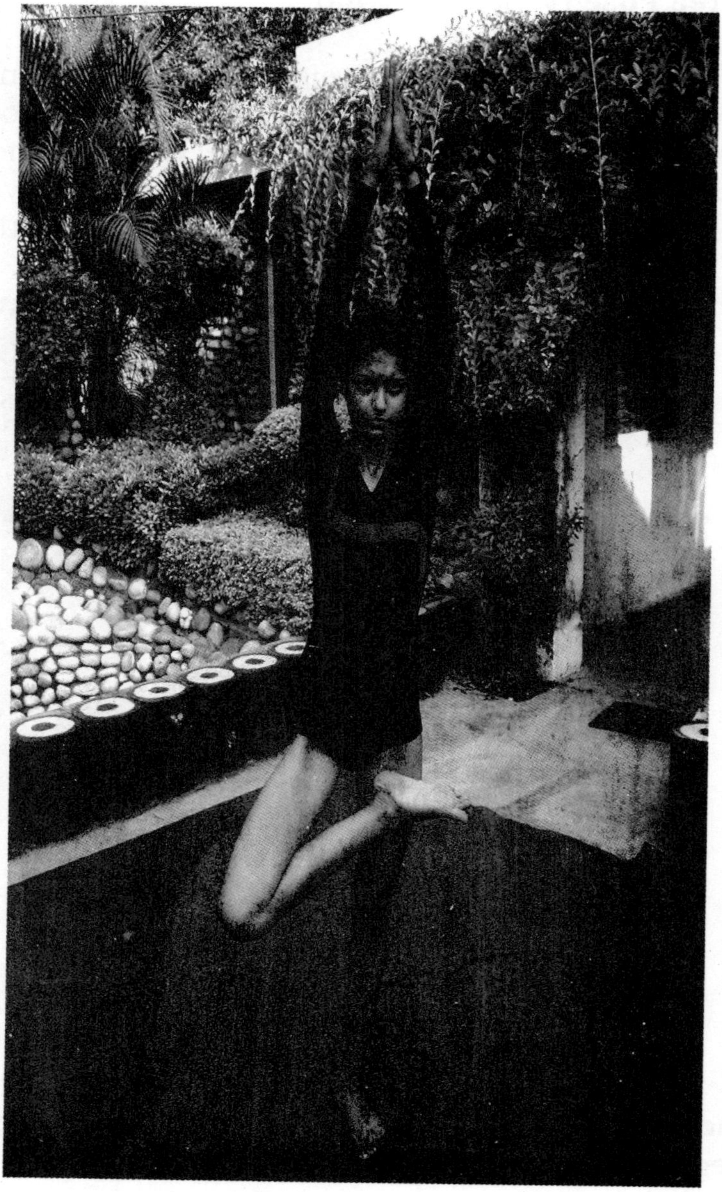

(Position-2)

and have many benefits such as health, strength, flexibility, concentration and grace.

Garuda Posture

Garuda with body of a man and the head, wings and claws of an eagle is a posture to warm-up and strengthen the whole body. Stand straight

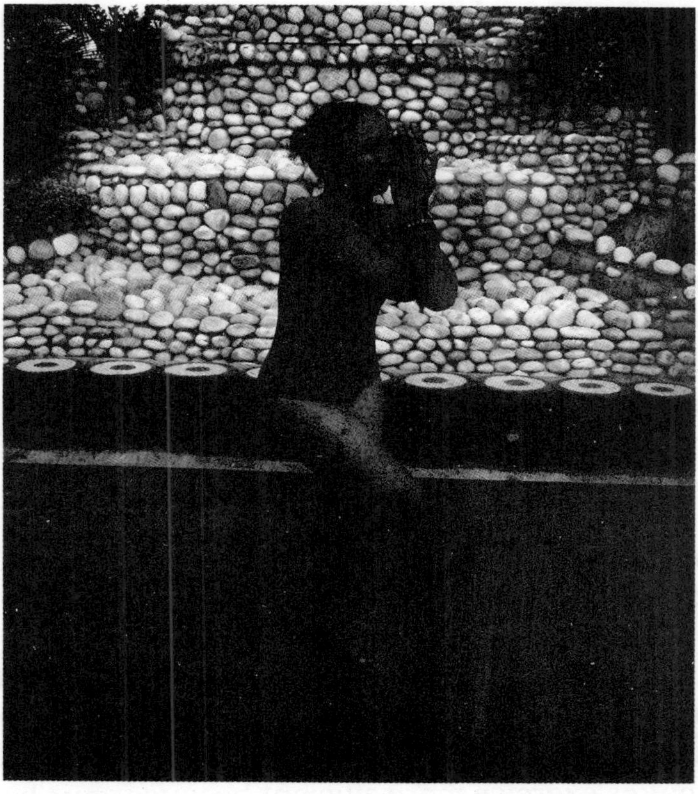

looking ahead. Bend your knees placing your left leg over around the right and simultaneously

tone the abdominal organs, cures irregular or faulty menstruation in females, stimulates endocrine glands, has curative and corrective effects on the disorders of joints, spinal cord, lungs, place your one arm over and around the other. Repeat the pose on the other leg having 10-12 counts on each side. This exercise relieves cramps in the calves.

Exercise Based on *Mantra* – *'No pain, much gain'*

The exercise should be done with the mantra 'No pain, much gain'. Life is meant to be comfortable, healthy and happy. And exercise should leave you feeling fresh and ready to work, not willing and ready for bed. From physical exercise one gets lightness, a capacity for work, firmness, tolerance of difficulties, elimination of impurities and stimulation of digestion. Exercising at a comfortable level leaves you feeling restless and shaky.

Comfortable Level – Avoid Strain and Pain Exercises

It is 50% of your maximum capacity. If you can walk for one hour, go for 30 minutes. If you can run for 30 minutes, cut it down to 15 minutes. It makes exercise more efficient because your body does not have to repair itself afterwards. Each woman has her own exercising threshold. If you have bursts of energy but tire quickly, go for very light exercises or walking. In winter, choose an indoor activity as extreme cold makes breathing difficult. Many men and women enroll themselves in a gym, but discontinue within few days after attending few sessions when they find the sessions too grueling and find waking in the morning feeling drained, aching all over, even depressed. Remember, your needs are exercising at comfortable level helping you progress steadily and keep your motivation high. If you are extremely overweight (say about 25 kg or above your standard weight) or have bad knees, do not run, walk or do lungs as these weight-bearing exercises, which cause strain and pain your joints even more. Instead, go for 30 minutes stationary cycling. It doesn't put pressure on your knees and ankles and stimulate the synovia fluid in your body, which lubricates the joints. There are various exercises, which stretch to a flexible body as described below:

Stretch for the Back

Lie on your stomach. Stretch your hand to hold the folded legs. Remain in this position. Push legs backwards, and raise upper body as much as you can (as shown in the illustration). Breathe deeply. Repeat this posture (known as Bow Posture) three to four times, which helps tone the abdominal organs, cures irregular or faulty menstruation in females, stimulates endocrine

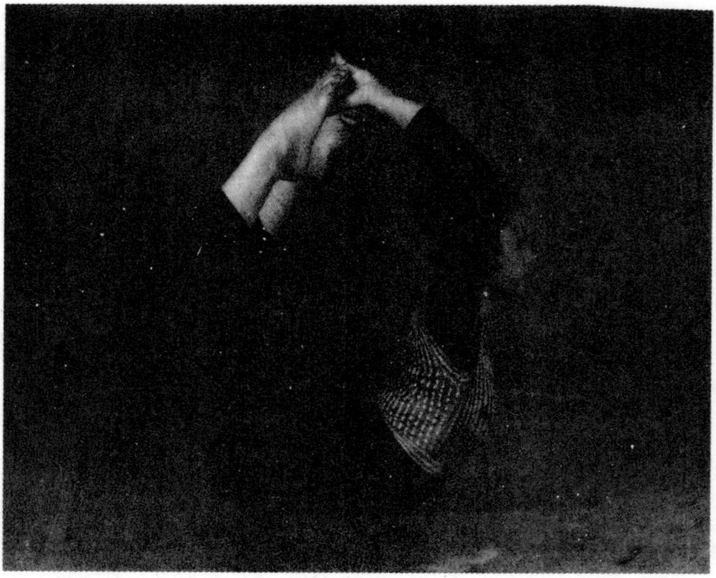

glands, has curative and corrective effects on the disorders of joints, spinalcord, lungs. Breathe deeply. Repeat this posture (known as Bow Posture) three to four times, which helps to chests, breasts and prevents fat from forming around stomach and hips.

Stretch for the Shoulders

This exercise has three positions. Stand straight and raise your arms opposite. Hold for 10 to 15 seconds. Now raise your arms straight over the head. Hold for 10 to 15 seconds. Finally bring both hands on sides parallel to the ground. Hold for 10 to 15 seconds. *This is a light exercise suggested during the pregnancy*, which keeps body in order without harming fetus. The exercise also

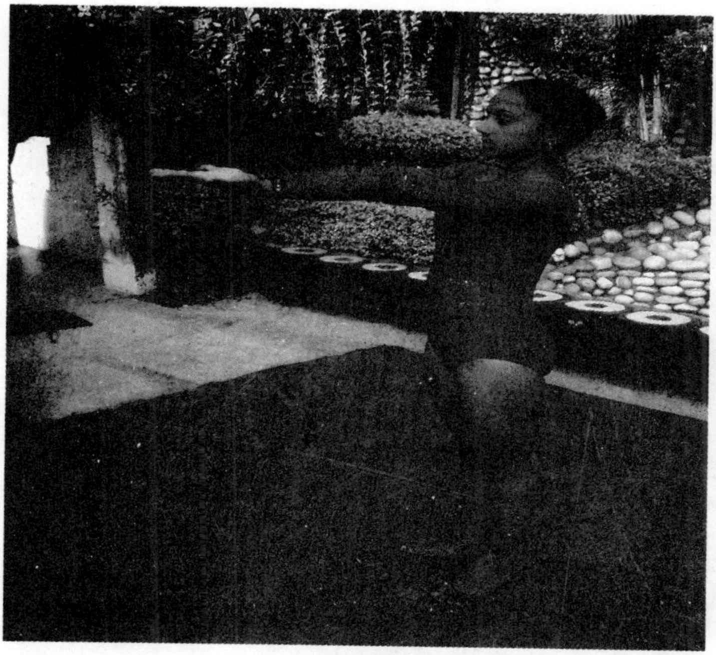

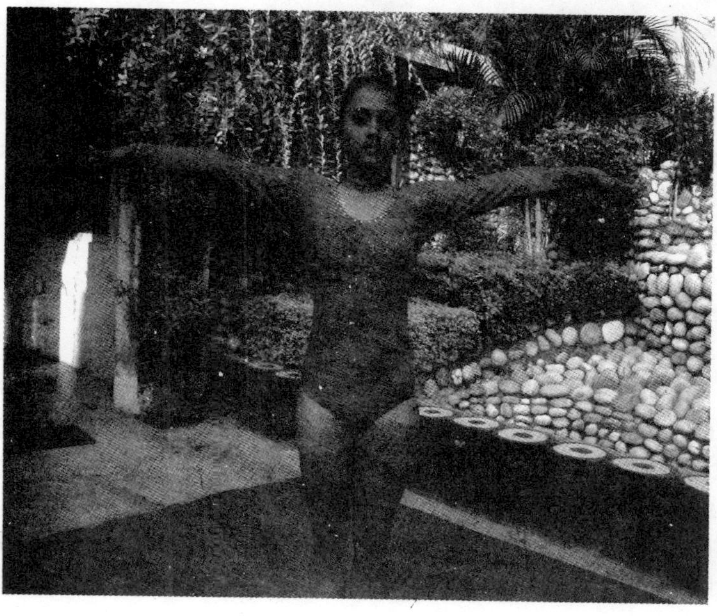

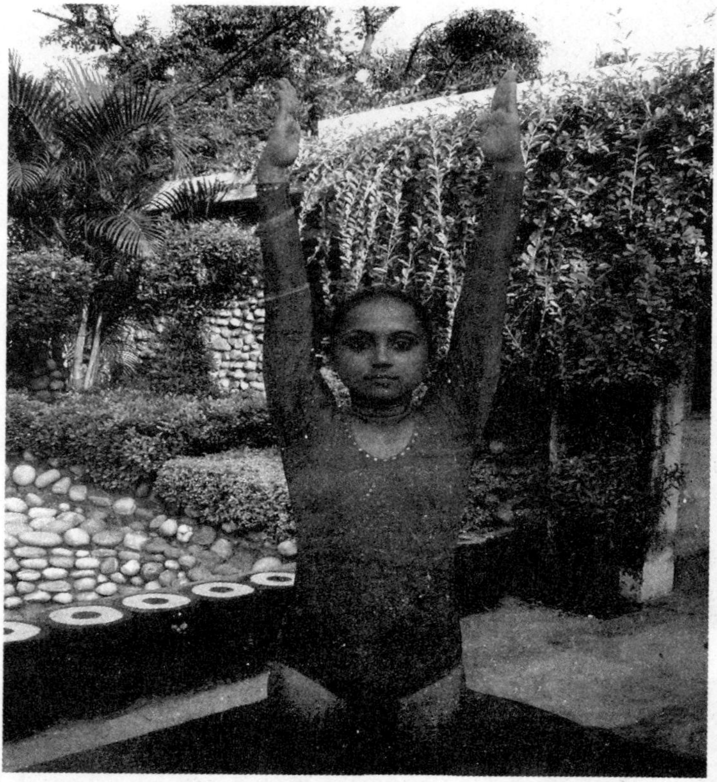

has strengthening effect upon shoulders, lungs and chest, and respiration system. It helps those who wish to add a few inches to their height.

For Stretching Hips and Thighs

Lie on stomach with chin or forehead touching the ground. Stretch the arms on sides of the body. Inhale, tense the arms, clench the fists tightly. Raise the legs as high as possible. Hold the position for few seconds retaining breath and lower the legs. Repeat exercise three to four times. The exercise has excellent effect on the muscles of hips, thighs, back and abdomen. It leaves beneficial effects on the digestive organs, cures constipation and cleans the kidneys. In case of difficulty to raise both legs, practice with simplified posture by raising one leg at a time.

Stretch Exercise for Tummy

Legs apart, raise arms over head, lower arms gradually to the waistline, stretching to the further, lowering them to touch the ground. Now place your palms on the ground and rest the crown

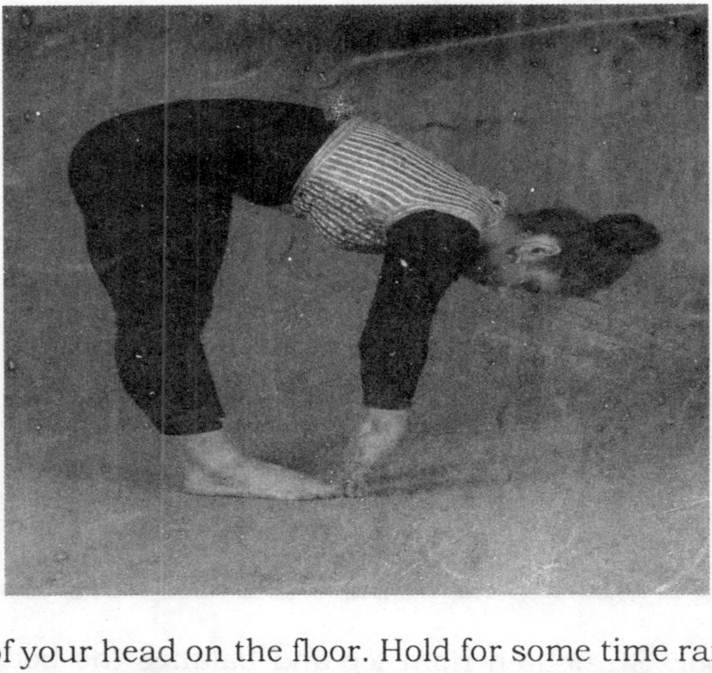

of your head on the floor. Hold for some time raise your head. This exercise removes fatigue, improves arches, relieve cramps in the calves and cures genital disorders including menstruation problems in females.

Stretching Waist

Spread legs two to three feet apart, arms sideways. Bend right knee, raising left leg off the

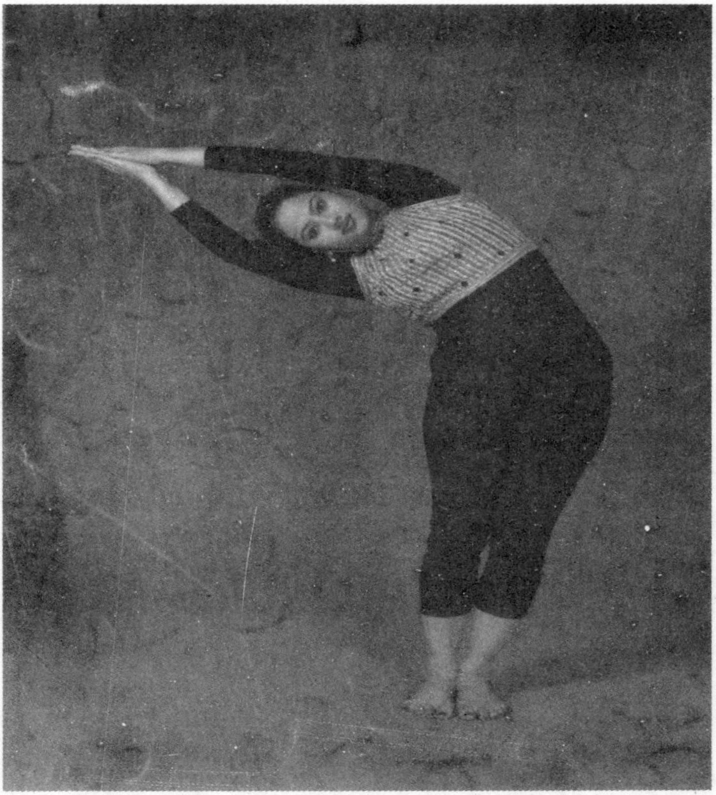

floor. Straighten right leg and balance the body. Return to initial position and repeat the posture to other side. This posture is known as Half-Moon Position and slims down the waist, hips and lower back. It softens up the spinal column and pelvic region.

Golden Rules of the Mind-Body Fitness

Don't just work on slimming your hips or toning your butt. You should be prepared for body-mind fitness. The savvy new age experts don't suggest instant weight loss as various health clubs and slimming centers usually claim. Instant weight loss or inch loss techniques simply divide bodies. There is need of a strong, toned and healthy mind-body. Here are few tips for mind-body fitness, which should be worked out four to five times a week:

1. The right breathing and right posture: can work wonders for your output. The idea is to do the right things with the right technique.
2. If you are making a day plan, try 15-20 minutes of cardio and 15-20 minutes of weight training each day.
3. If you are making a weekly programme, keep three days for cardio, stretching and strengthening, and other two days for weights.
4. A casual walk after lunch or dinner or a climb up the stairs should be a daily routine for everyone (except during periods, pregnancy and post-natal period).

5. Be careful about your cardio workouts. The wrong twist or move could hurt you. Especially after general exercise routine or aerobics.
6. Go by the needs of your body. If you do weights thrice a week, keep two days for the upper body (back, shoulders, chest and arms) and one day for the lower body (calves, thighs and hips)
7. An essential workout is a balanced mix of cardiovascular exercises, weight training and meditation.
8. Always warm up prior to your workout. Set aside minutes for a cool-down, even if you are in hurry.
9. It is good to have some water before a workout, sips in between and enough of it half an hour after.
10. The floor where you are exercising has to be appropriate. It is best to have carpeted or soft wooden flooring. Concrete flooring will harm your joints.
11. Wear the right footwear for the activity.
12. Eat well. It is a vital to fitness. Cut down on fried foods, sweets and colas.
13. If you don't get your eight-hour sleep, you cannot aspire to fitness.
14. Think positive because the ideal body is never possible. It is more important to be comfortable with yourself.
15. At least initially, exercise under a trained expert to avoid injury.
16. Avoid to jog.

Mind-Body Workout

This posture is known as Cow-head position which activates muscles of entire body, tones up

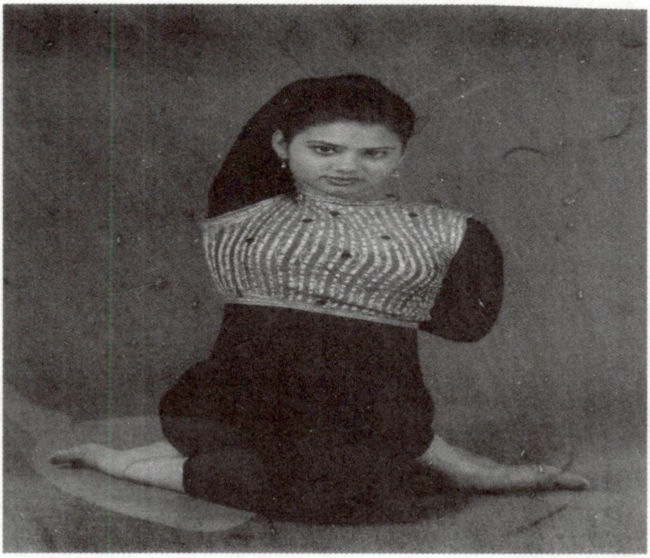

the joint muscles and nerves, restores the synovial fluid (a joint fluid in the body), strengthens the lungs and heart and helps bust development during teenage and period of pregnancy. To practice this exercise, sit on the floor. Fold left leg in and right leg over the left leg so that one knee lies over the other. Take left arm on the back placing left hand between shoulder blades. Now take right hand behind on the back and hook fingers with the fingers of left hand. Sit in this position for 30 seconds and interchange the position of legs and arms.

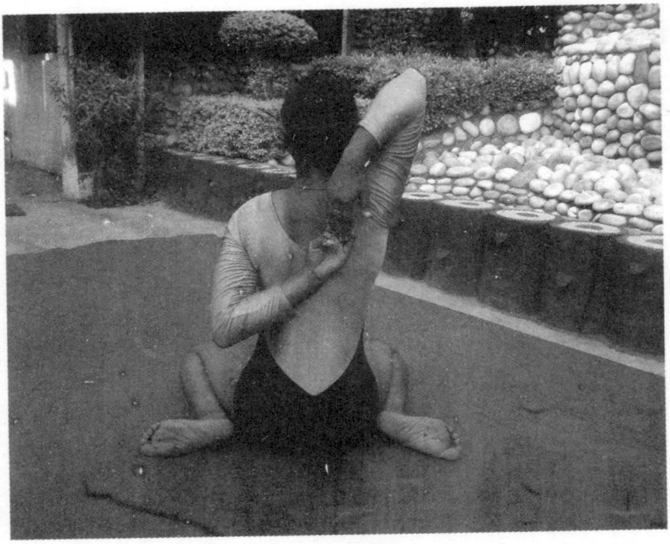

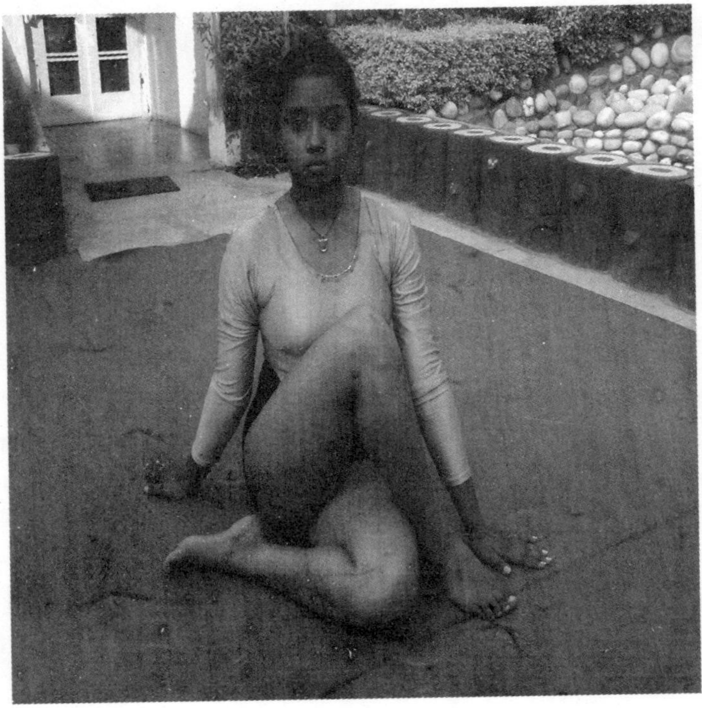

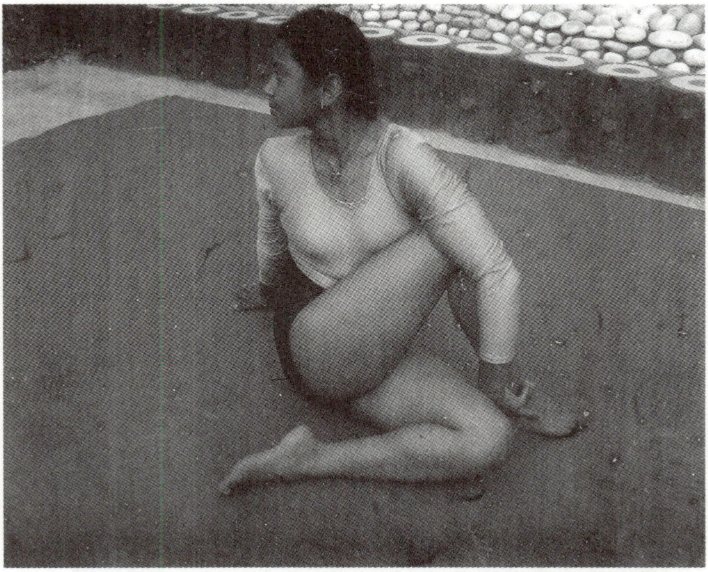

If You Go to a Gym

Go in for cardio-vascular exercises such as kickboxing, steps, the recumbent cycle and the Swiss ball. You could also opt for outdoor sports like tennis, squash or swimming. But avoid jogging on roads, you will have to pay its price later on above the age of 45 when you will find weakness in joints and body strength. We do not have the hormones that allow for increased muscle mass. Weights increase the muscle tissues in human body, which causes weight gain. This also means a cut in your fat percentage, since muscle tissues help you burn more calories even as you sit or stand.

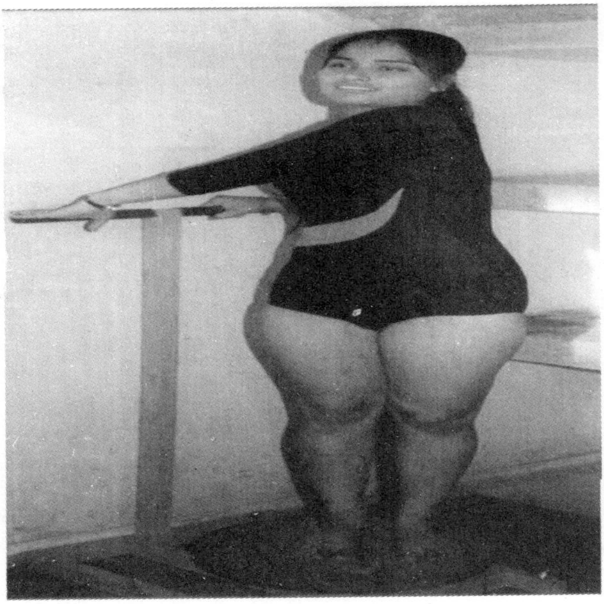

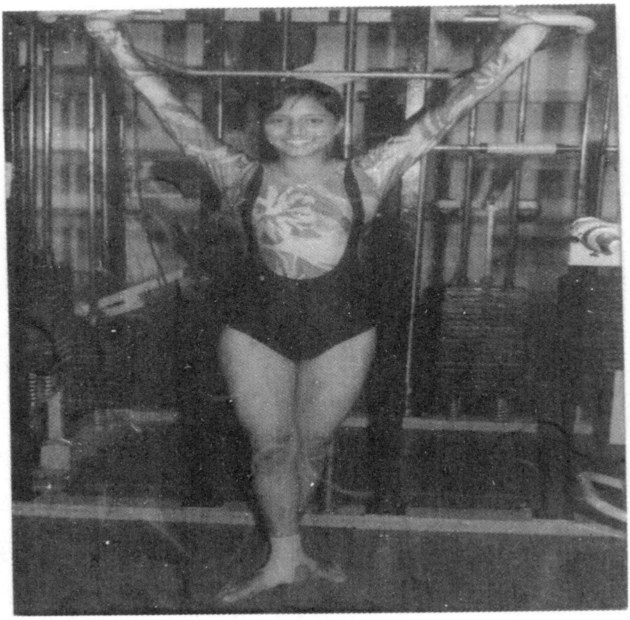

A Powerful Tool to Strengthen Bones

Mind-Body workout helps the bones of the body a powerful tool against osteoporosis, which increases chances of wrist, feet, hip and spine fracture. Beware of hurting yourself if you work without an instructor in a gym. It is also important to work with the right kind of equipment otherwise you might end up with problems of the lower back, spinal cord, elbow and shoulder joints. Remember, warm-ups are important when working out with weights as well. One important part of the body that we ignore is the spine. Stretching, strengthening and exercises like cobra and tortoise posture are helpful.

Cobra Posture

Lie on your stomach. Raise your trunk off the floor and throw your head-back. This exercise helps to tone up spinal column, activates

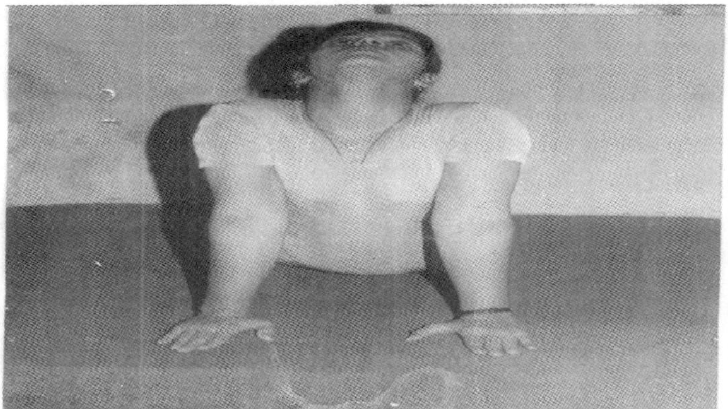

abdominal area, leaves beneficial effect on adrenal glands, stimulate digestion and soothes backaches.

Tortoise Posture

This posture improves circulation of spinal column and the pelvic region. To do this exercise, wide your legs as much as you can sideways, one leg at a time. Tighten the muscles of your leg and

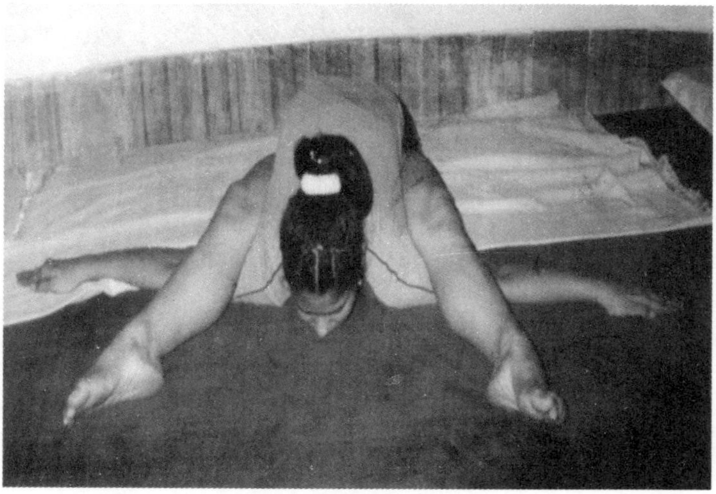

(Position-1)

keep toes pointing upwards. Sit erect, hook big toes with your index and middle fingers. Now bend forward and rest your forehead and chin on the floor as shown in illustration. This exercise is especially beneficial for females and helps to keep joint, muscles, organs and nerves strong and healthy. This exercise also improves circulation in the pelvic region, makes hamstring muscles

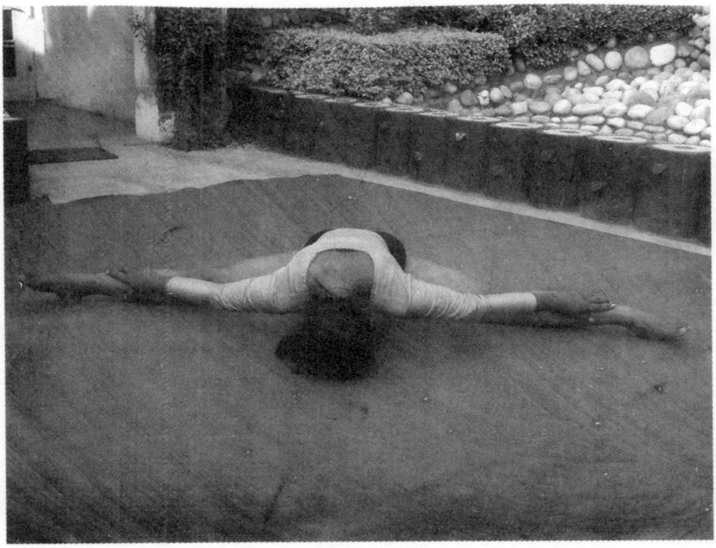

(Position-2)

elastic, cures menstruation disorders of women, strengthen genital organs and increases sex power. In case of difficulty to do, it can be performed on single leg also.

And Finally Relax !

Do not forget to mediate and relax. Meditation posture and Complete Relaxation Posture (*Shavasana*) help to relax different parts of your body. You could cool down with stretching or five minutes of cardio to slow your metabolism rate and to bring down the body temperature. In Sanskrit *shava* means 'corpse' in which one lies on the back like a corpse with relaxed mind and body. In this posture keep arms at the sides, legs stretched out slightly apart, eyes closed, breath

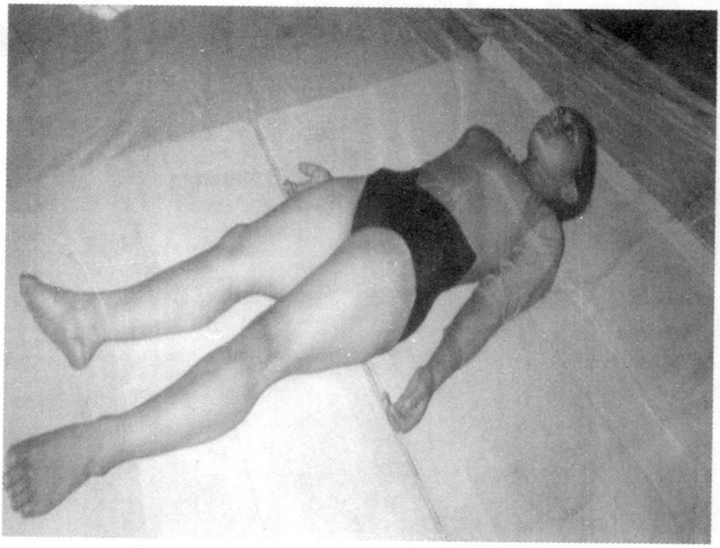

rhythmical slowly and deeply. Keep the brain completely empty. This exercise cures high blood pressure, insomnia, nervous disorder, relieve depression, eliminate the toxins accumulating in the blood, recharge energy and regenerate body cells.

Don't Neglect Arms and Feet

Exercising Arms: Lie down on the floor, face downwards and place the hands on the ground directly below the shoulders. Raise the body from the ground without allowing the body to sag. Weight of the body should be supported on the toes and hands. Hold for as much time as you can. Lower the body on the ground. Inhale as the body lowered, exhale as the body is raised.

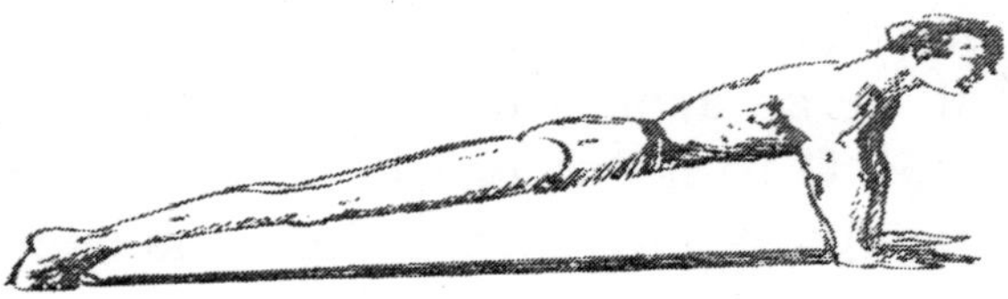

Developing the Muscles of Upper Arms: Stand erect, heels together, knees straight. Raise the arms upward on a level with the shoulders. Clench the fists, flex the arms contracting the biceps strongly and drop the fists downwards to the

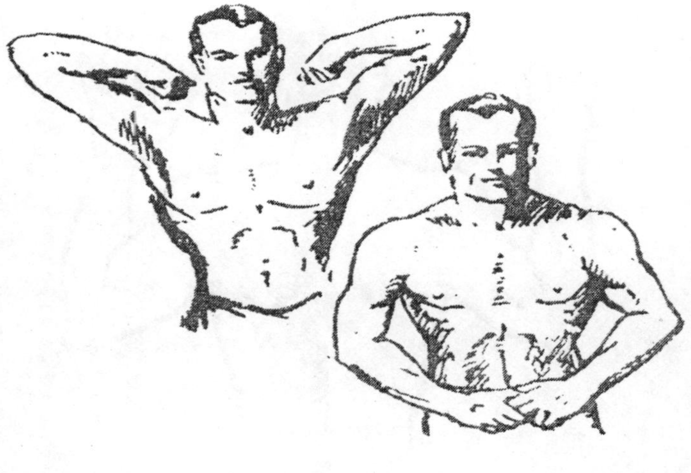

shoulders by slightly raising the upper arms. Then lower the arms contracting the muscles of the upper ribs, and grip the hands in front of the abdomen. Hold. Repeat few times. On completion of the exercise drop the arms to the sides and relax. Inhale as arms raised, exhale as the arms are lowered. During exercise concentrate the mind on the biceps of the arms, the muscles on the ribs and muscles above the shoulders.

Developing the Muscles of Hands and Wrists: Stand erect, knees straight, heels together, feet turned outwards, arms raised from the sides, elbows bent and hands at the height of head. Clench the left fist tightly, at the same time open the right hand vigorously to the full extent of the fingers. Repeat by clenching and opening each

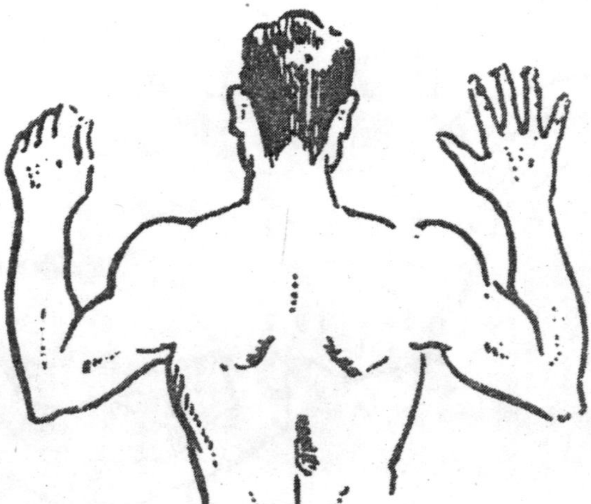

hand alternately. On completion of the exercise, lower the arms to the sides and relax.

Strengthening the Ankles and Developing the Muscles of the Shins: Sit on a chair. Raise the feet from the floor keeping the knees straight. Circle both feet slowly inward towards each other, pointing the toes and raising the feet upwards to the utmost extent.Now reverse the movement by

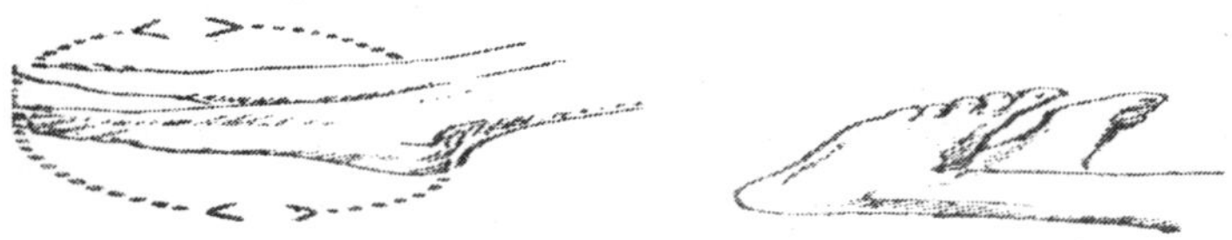

circling both feet slowly outwards from each other and raising the feet upwards to the utmost extent. On completion of the exercise relax. Breathe normal. During the exercise concentrate the mind on the contracted muscles on the fronts and sides of the shins. For development of the muscles of the shins, turn the feet slowly upwards to the fullest extent contracting the muscles on the fronts of the shins as shown in the sketch. During the exercise concentrate the mind on the contracted muscles.

14

Power Yoga for Weight Loss

Power Yoga or *Ashtanga Yoga* is believed to be the original postures designed by Patanjali, the sage who initiated Yoga over 300 years ago. The word Ashtanga in Sanskrit *Eight-fold Path.* 'Ashta' means eight and 'Anga' means limbs.

The Eight Limbs of Yoga

1. *Yama*: refers to Ahinsa (Non-violence), Satya (Truth), Asetya (Non-stealing), Brahmacharya (Self-control) and Aparigraha (Unselfishness).

2. *Niyama*: refers to Saucha (Cleanliness), Santosha (Contentment), Tapas (Effort), Svadhyaya (Self study) and Ishwara Pranidhama (Faith in God).

3. *Asana*: means posture.

4. *Pranayama*: means control of the senses such as taste, touch, smell, sight and hearing.

5. *Dharna*: means concentration.

6. *Dhyana*: means meditation.

7. *Samadhi*: means that unites with God.

8. *Yogasana*

The following rules should be kept in mind to practice Pranayama or a Yogasana:

1. Start practice at the age of eight to ten years.

2. Exercise is equally useful for both sexes: male and females.

3. Practice in a peaceful, calm, noiseless and airy environment.

4. Wear clothes, which are sufficient to protect the body. Avoid wearing tight clothes.

5. Practice empty stomach, two hours after breakfast and four hours after a meal and an hour after having a cup of tea or coffee.

6. Start practicing for short period and gradually increase the duration.

7. The practitioner should be a vegetarian as far as possible.

Yogic Breathing

These are of two types:

1. *Exhalation (Rechaka)*: Begin with the abdomen completely emptying the lungs. It is a wave like movement by abdominal, middle and upper parts of the chest.

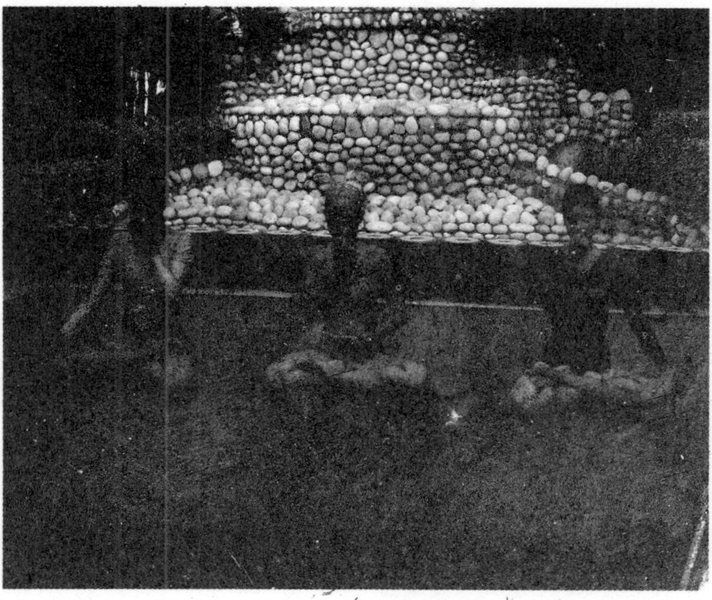

2. *Inhalation (Puraka)*: After exhalation, begin to inhale and fill the lungs. The whole process of inhaling and exhaling should be done as one smooth, continuous movement like a wave.

Benefits

It is important for good health and should be regarded as a gift from the nature.

1. Brings respiratory organs into play and guard against pulmonary infections.

2. Prevents asthma and heart trouble.

3. Nourishes vital organs, endocrine glands, nervous centers and body tissues.

4. Maintains blood pressure in the arteries.

5. Calms nervous system.

6. Provides mental and physical peace.

Before Practicing Yoga

Following are some useful tips:

1. Warming up exercise is essential before starting Yoga practice for slimming and shaping figure, and to obtain perfect results. Brisk walk in the fresh morning air is very beneficial. Brisk walk gives exercise to whole body, especially useful for hips and thighs.

2. Always cool down after a yoga session with slow, gentle stretches. When you begin to feel more poised, loose limbed, coordinated, stretched and toned, feel like as if you are gliding rather walking.

3. If you are extremely overweight, about 20 kg or above your standard weight or have strain, pain and inflammation in joint —do not run, walk or do lunges. These weight bearing exercises strain your joints even more.

4. Pre-exercise meal should be light. Practice at least two hours after a meal.

5. Cool down after exercising a session with slow and gentle stretches.

6. Consult a doctor or a yoga teacher before embarking on an yogic exercise programme, especially when you are above 45 years of age or you have a personal or family history of high blood pressure or heart problem.

7. Too much and too fast yogic practice does not provide instant results — these simply lead to injuries, aches and pains.

Power Yoga

It is a combination of dynamic breathing and strong, flowing movement, which creates a high-heat, high-energy workout. Yoga programme helps flow energy into the body, build strength, release tension from tight joints and loosening muscles.

Based on the classical and original yoga system called *Ashtanga*, Power yoga is a complete mind and body workout that develops concentration and reduces stress. Power yoga goes beyond the relaxation and marches towards health and fitness. One of the essential principles of Ashtanga yoga is *tapas* or heat — the more you sweat, the better it is. The heat releases tension and stiffness from the muscles making them more pliable. The heat / perspiration process expedite the release of toxins from the body and also intensify an inner spiritual fire within body.

The structure of Power Yoga or Ashtanga makes you repeatedly go through the postures beneficial to trim the body. If you do the right poses in the right order, the mind and body are cleansed of toxins. Don't overdo exercises, else you could put undue strain on your muscles and joints. The exercise must be done in a series, under the guidance of a qualified yoga teacher. These poses balance the different areas of the body and improve circulation. The nervous system is purified and strengthened and the body is realigned. Shava Asana performed at the end of the sequence allows the body to return back to its normal metabolic state. It enables the body and mind to be in a state of complete relaxation.

Overweight Teenagers

Girls between the age of 14 to 18 tend to put on excess weight, largely because their bodies are undergoing natural changes around this time. Women, face this problem after their first baby.

Obesity is disastrous for women looking for a career. It becomes a real mental burden for those afflicted with it. Even if the problem does not cause to physical health, its psychological effect can be far more damaging. Remember, slimming can be done without tears by practicing yogic exercises regularly. To maintain a perfect, the amount of energy you consume must be equal to the amount of energy you burn.

Obesity has become a worldwide health hazard for majority of people — male and female of every age. There is a difference between obesity and overweight. Overweight is not obesity, but every obese person is overweight. It has been observed that an obese person loses average two to three kilograms of weight every month to fight obesity practicing a few selected yogic postures supported by a balanced and proper diet. *Surya Namaskar Asana* (Sun Exercise) has been recommended to fight overweight and stimulate the muscles of whole body.

This asana involves various bending forward and backward movements. The routine will begin with the practice of Surya Namaskar to stretch and strengthen all major muscles of the body and also to improve blood circulation to specific organs, replenishing them with fresh oxygen and nutrients, followed by exercises to strengthen the upper and lower body and also the abdominal muscles; thereby making it a complete fitness routine. The posture has ten positions as described below with illustrations:

Position 1: Stand with your weight evenly

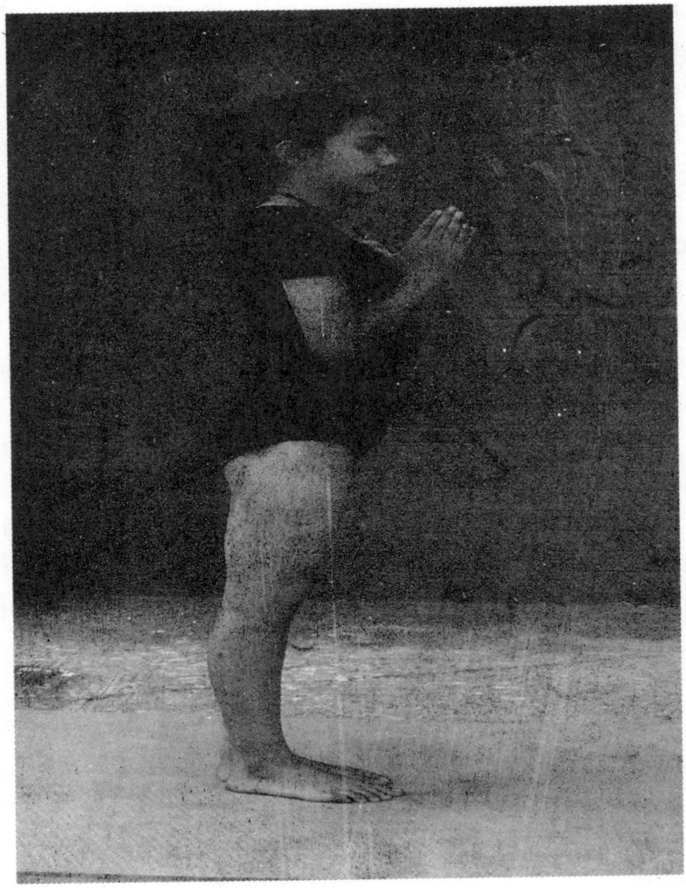

(Position-1)

distributed and your back straight. Exhale as you put your palms together in the 'prayer pose'.

Position 2: Inhale as you stretch your arms back so that your hips move forward, your back arches and your head is tilted back.

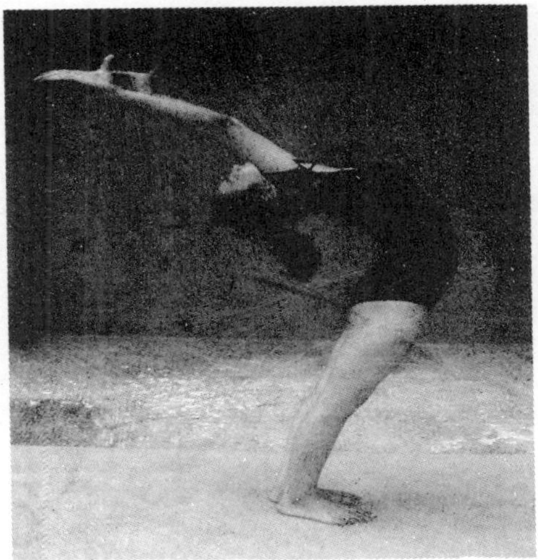

(Position-2)

Position 3: Inhale as you extend your left leg behind you, resting the knee on the ground.

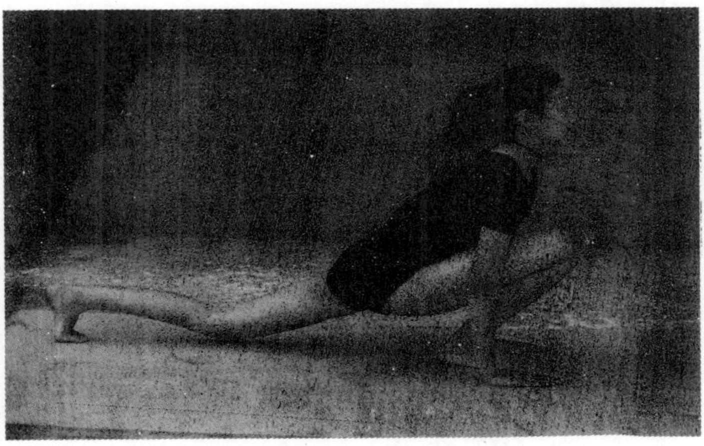

(Position-3)

Position 4: Exhale as you extend your right leg too and hold your breath as you push yourself

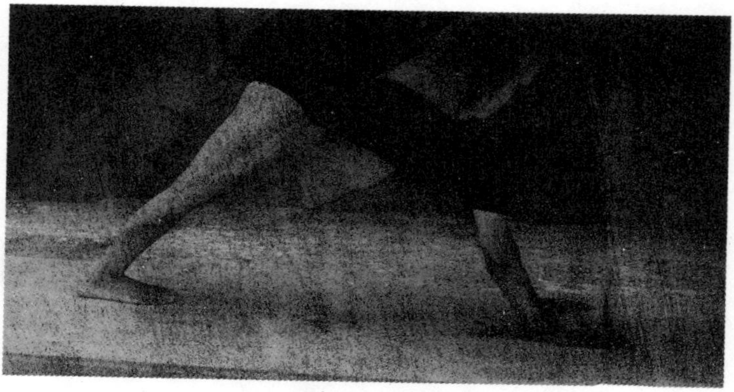

(Position-4)

up on your feet. Raise your hips so that your body forms an inverted 'V'.

Position 5: Exhale as you lower your knees, chest and chin on the floor. The hips are off the floor.

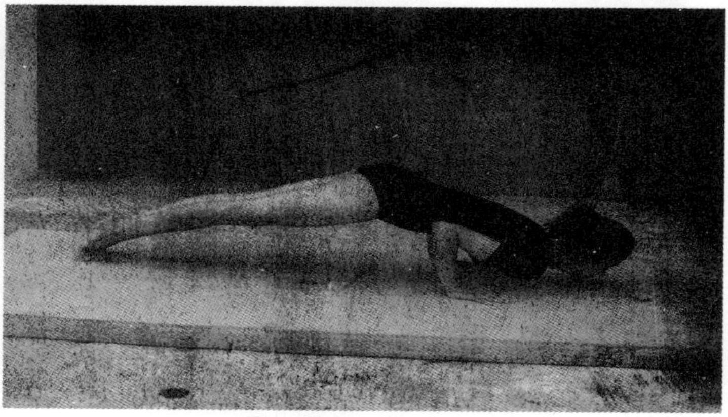

(Position-5)

Position 6: Raise head, trunk, hips, thighs and knees from floor.

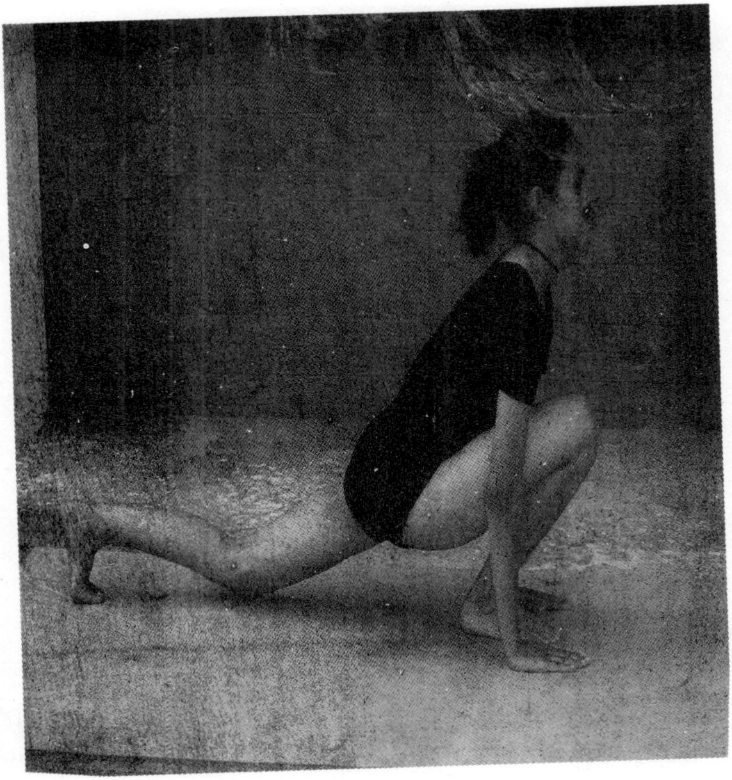

(Position-6)

Position 7: Inhale as you move your left foot forward between your hands, allowing your right knee to bend to the floor, and look up. Left leg remains stretched.

Position 8: Raise the body with hands backward.

Position 9: Bend backward with raised hands and feet joined.

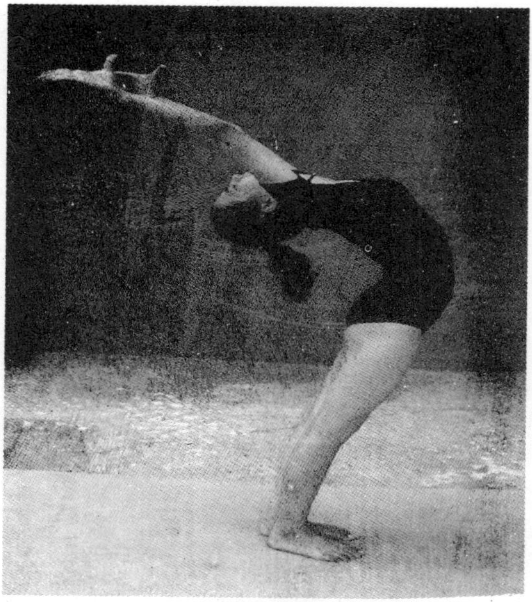

(Position-9)

Position 10: Return to the original standing position with folded hands.

Yoga Postures to Stimulate the Muscles of Face and Upper Portion of Body

Ushtra Asana and Natraj Asana are recommended yogic exercises as described below with illustrations:

Viparitakarani (Inverted Posture) : In Sanskrit Viparita means inverted and karani means action.

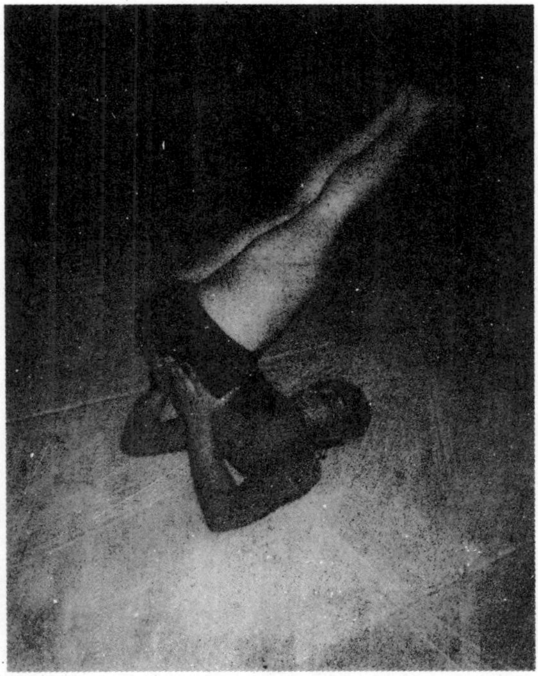

Lie on the back. Inhale. Raise legs and hips with the help of hands. Exhale. The legs should form angle of 60-70 degree. Lower the legs gently on the ground. Relax. Repeat exercise three to four times. If you suffer from high blood pressure, consul a doctor before doing this posture. This posture is beneficial for reviving the body, prevents formation of facial wrinkles, regenerates thyroid and pituitary glands, control nervous system and increase flow of blood to neck, throat and head.

Ushtra Asana (Camel Posture): This asana helps remove stiffness in the neck and shoulders, cures visionary and voice defects, throat troubles, tonsils, chronic headache and respiratory system.

The asana activates the facial tissues and strengthen the muscles of chin and neck. The

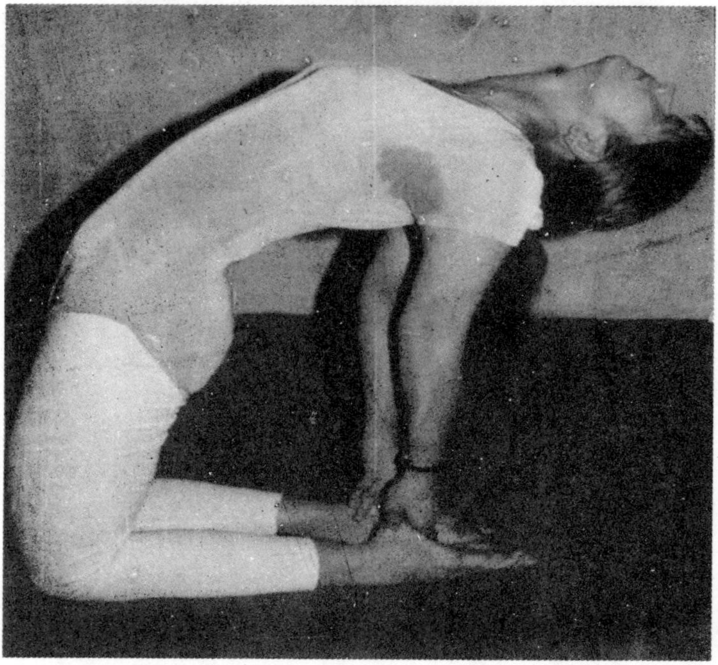

posture enhance facial and neck beauty and cure double chin.

Natraj Asana: This asana is dedicated to Lord Shiva. As a cosmic dancer, Shiva is called God of Dances. This posture generates vigor, vitality, potency, flexibility to the limbs, shoulders and hip joints, strengthens the major bones of the body, enhances digestive power, leaves good effect on the spine, removes spinal rigidity rid the body from extra fat. Stay in the position as shown in

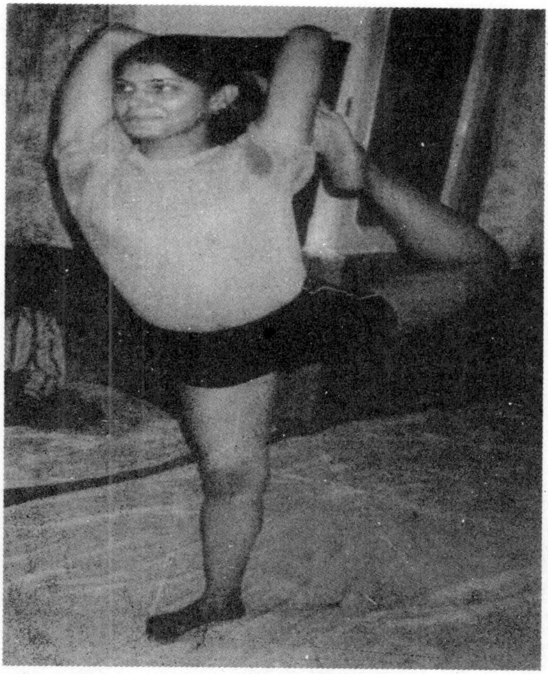

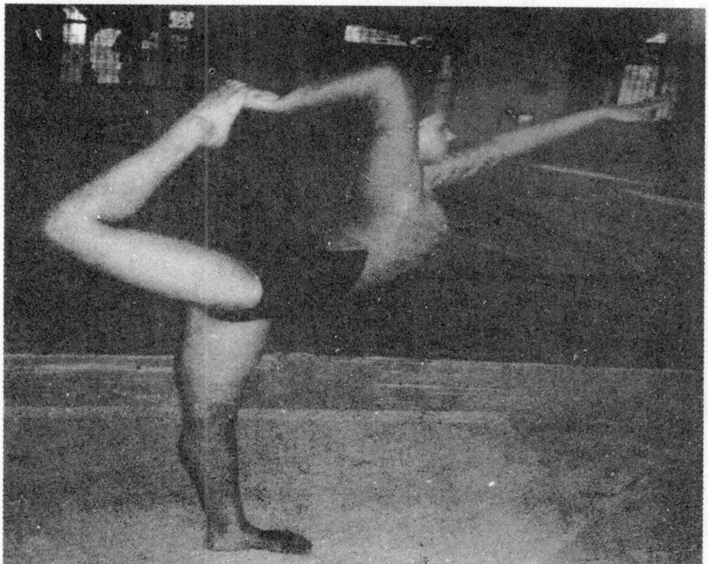

illustration for 8-10 seconds and keep breathing normal. Perform posture on both legs: left and then on right leg. Make four to six rounds daily.

Yoga Posture for Slimming Back

Sit in Yog Mudra (The symbol of Yoga). To do this asana, sit in the Padmasana position keeping the spinal column upright. Place hands behind the back and grab the wrist of one hand with the other hand. Now lean forward gently

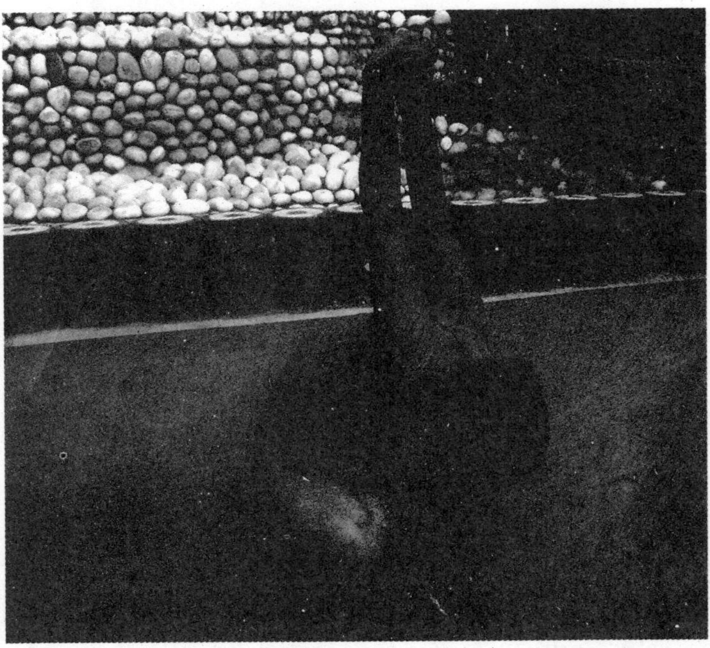

without straining or jerking the spinal column. The therapeutic advantages of this asana include remedy for constipation, tone up the abdominal

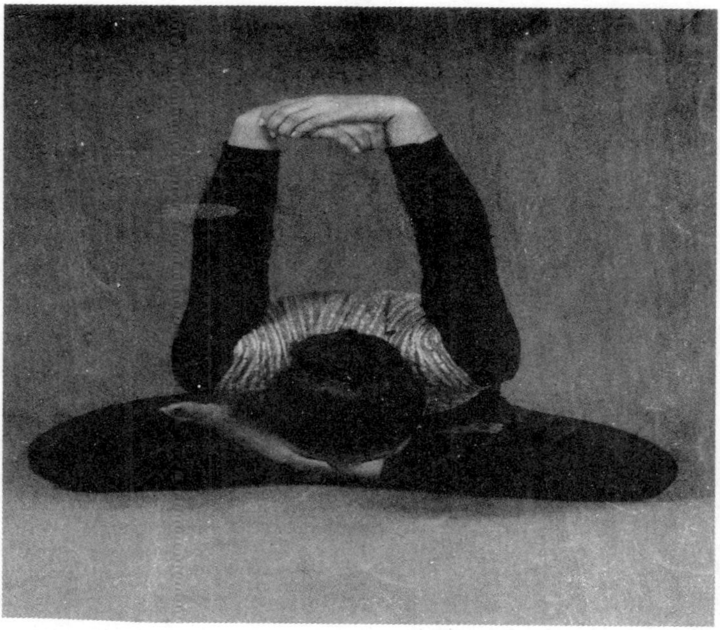

muscles/organs, exercise lungs, leave curative effect for asthmatics, strengthen the digestive system, enhance sexual potentiality, remove extra fatness from thighs, hips, back and arms.

Yoga Posture to Relieve Fatness on Hips

Hal Asana (Plough Posture): To do this asana, lie on the back, arms stretched by the side. Raise legs slowly stretched vertically. Then lower the legs behind the head until the tips of the feet touch the ground. Remain in this position for 25-40 seconds breathing regularly. Return to the starting position. Relax and repeat the posture four to five times. Besides relieving fatness on hips, this posture helps relieve digestive problems,

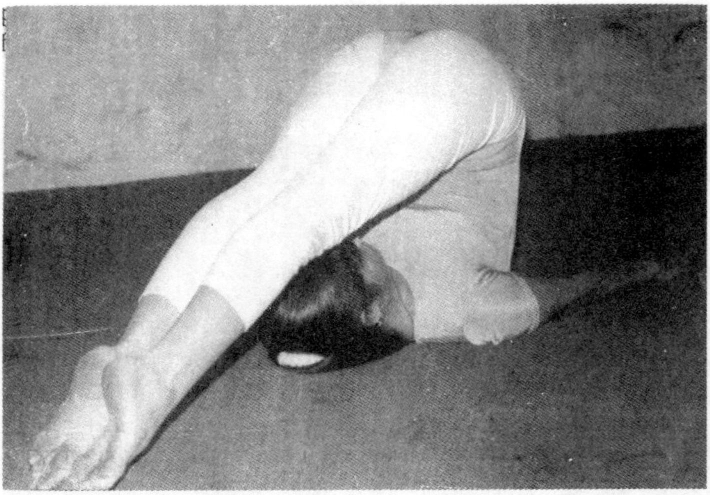

increases supply of blood to facial muscles and head, prevent fat from forming on stomach, waist, spine and back. This asana have regenerating effect on the glandular system, clears menstrual disorders and removes exhaustion and fatigue.

Vajroli Mudra (Boat Posture): This balancing pose strengthens thighs, hips and abdominal

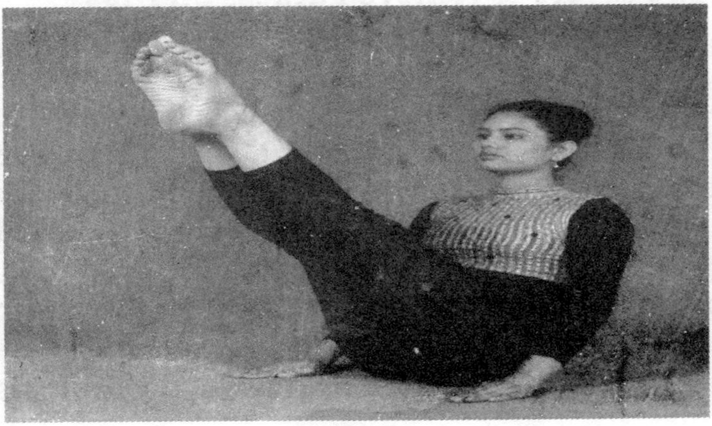

muscles. The asana rids the digestive organs of toxins and helps to develop the sex will-power in men and women between the age 20 to 40.

Yoga Posture to Shed Off Fat Around Stomach, Waist and Trunk

Perform *Supta Vajra Asana* to melt fatness around waist especially after childbirth. This Supine Pelvic Posture also strengthens male and female sex organs. Sit between the heels not on them as Muslims sit for their *'Namaz'*. Lean

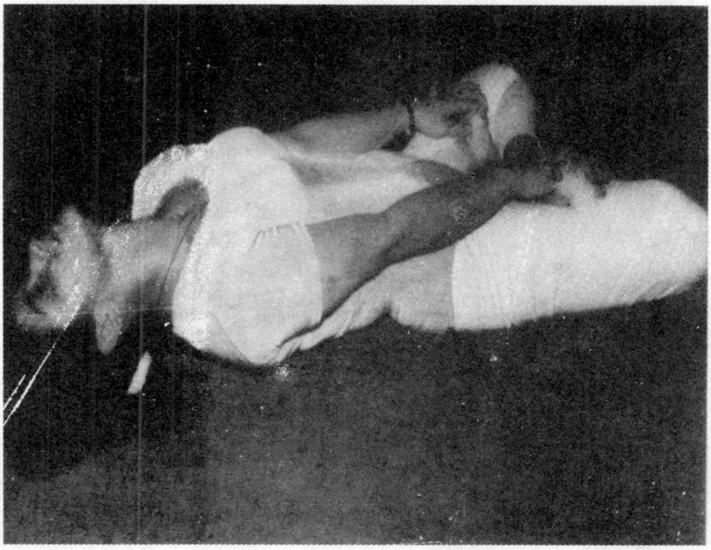

backward slowly until back of the head rest on the ground, placing hands under the nape of neck. Relax for 6-8 seconds, then return to Vajra Asana. Repeat exercise for four to five times.

Yoga Posture to Slim Abdomen

Practice *Mayur Asana ((Peacock Posture*). To do this posture, kneel on the ground, knees apart, palms flat on the floor, fingers pointing

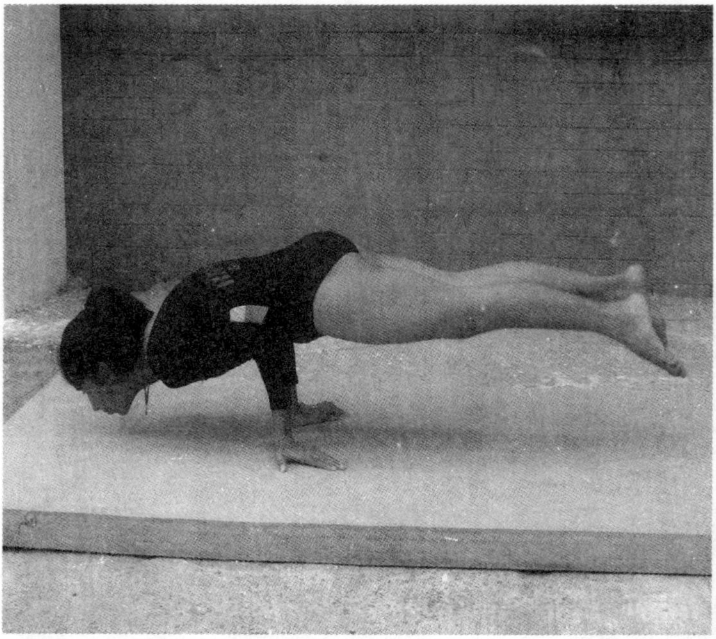

towards the face, elbows under the abdomen just under the navel. Lean forward to touch the ground with forehead and stretching out the leg behind raising the feet and head. Keep body horizontal (parallel to the ground). Stay balanced on the arms as long as possible, then lie down on stomach. This posture tones up abdominal muscles, cures constipation, brings the body into equilibrium and fortifies the hands, wrists and forearms.

Yoga Posture for Slimming Legs, Knees, Ankles and Thighs

Vir Bhadra Asana (Warrior Pose) comprises of three positions as shown in illustrations. These exercises help increase stamina, improve balance and concentration, strengthen muscles of the chest, shoulders, back and stomach.

Position 1: Stand straight. Jump and spread legs 3-4 feet apart with arms sideways. Raise your arms

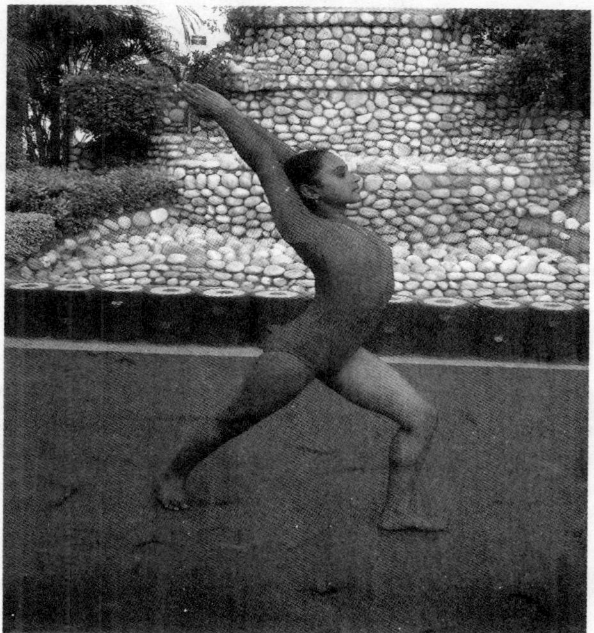

(Position-1)

up. Turn right foot out 90 degree and left in 45 degree. Revolve your hips and turn your trunk to the right. Look up. Return to initial position and repeat the pose on left side.

Position 2: Bend your right knees to form a right angle and look at your fingertips as shown in illustration.

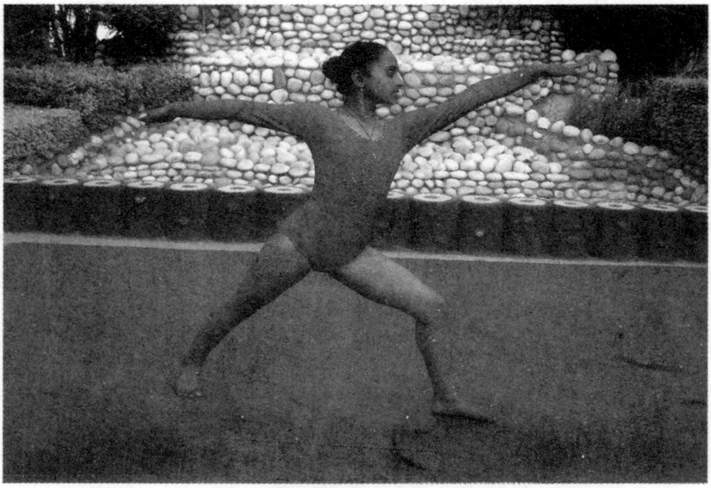

(Position-2)

Position 3: In this posture raise left leg off the floor. Straighten your right leg and balance on it as shown in illustration. Return to the original

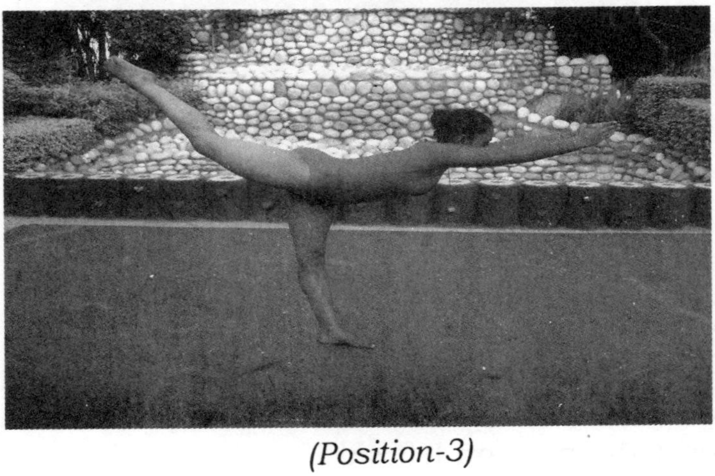

(Position-3)

position and repeat the pose on left leg. This asana builds stamina and improves balance and concentration.

Yoga Posture to Slim Arms, Hands and Wrists

Janusir Asana, Parivritta Janusir Asana and Janusir Merudanda Asana are best recommended

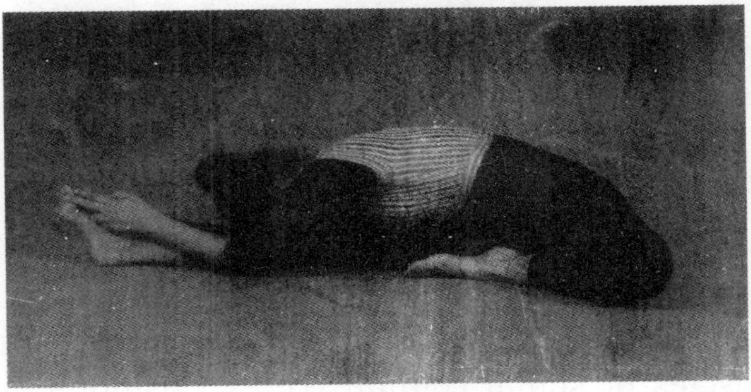

(Janusir Asana)

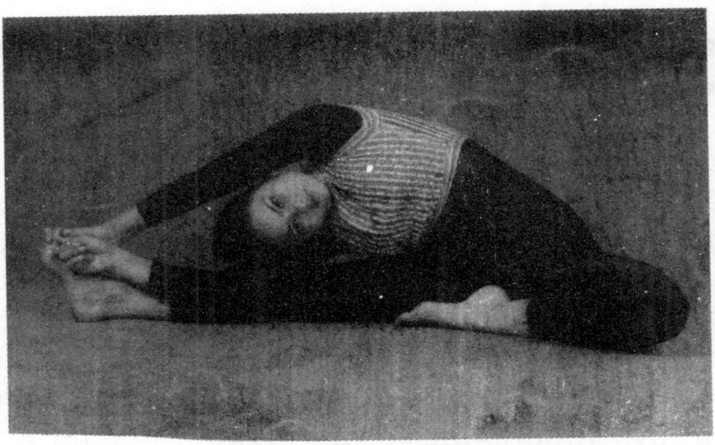

(Parivritta Janusir Asana)

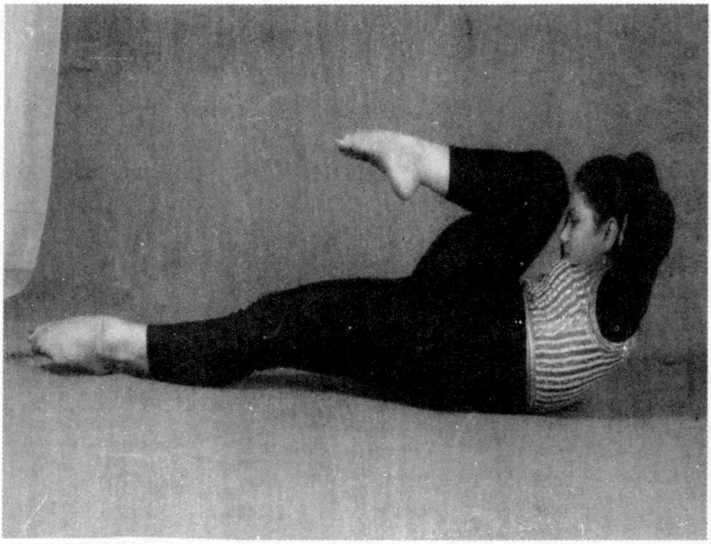

(Janusir Merudanda Asana)

positions for slimming and strengthen the muscles of spinal column. These positions are excellent for women.

Yoga Posture to Relieve Spinal Column Deformities

Sarvang Asana: Sarva means all and anga means parts. To do this asana, lie on your back. Bend your knees towards the chest. Raise your hips and legs off the floor supporting back with your palms. Straighten your legs perpendicular to the floor. This asana helps relieve headaches, cold, cough, constipation, enhance facial beauty and improve functioning of all organs, glands and nerves of face and upper part of body.

Recommended Slimming Yogic Routine for Beginners (30 minutes)

Warming up exercises	5 minutes
Surya Namaskar Asana	3 minutes
Ushtra Asana	2 minutes
Supta Vajra Asana	2 minutes
Sarvang Asana	2 minutes
Vir Bhadra Asana	4 minutes
Natraj Asana	2 minutes
Parivritta Janusir Asana (3 Positions)	3 minutes
Yog Mudra	2 minutes
Shava Asana	5 minutes

Recommended Slimming Routine for Children (15 minutes)

Warming up exercises	3 minutes
Surya Namaskar Asana	3 minutes
Vir Bhadra Asana	3 minutes
Supta Vajra Asana	1 minute
Yog Mudra	2 minutes
Shava Asana	3 minutes

Recommended Postures for Women (30 minutes)

Warming up exercises	3 minutes
Surya Namaskar Asana	4 minutes
Hal Asana	2 minutes
Ushtra Asana	2 minutes
Mayur Asana	1 minute

Sarvang Asana	2 minutes
Supta Vajra Asana	2 minutes
Parivritta Janusir Asana (3 minutes)	3 minutes

Recommended Yoga Routine for Pregnant (10 minutes)

Light Warming up exercises	2 minutes
Yog Mudra	1 minute
Meditation	1 minute
Parivritta Janusir Asana (3 Positions)	2 minutes
Shava Asana	4 minutes

Recommended Postures for Adults (30 minutes)

Warming up exercises	5 minutes
Hal Asana	2 minutes
Parivritta Janusir Asana (3 Positions)	3 minutes
Yog Mudra	2 minutes
Vajroli Mudra	2 minutes
Ushtra Asana	2 minutes
Viparitakarani	2 minutes
Sarvang Asana	2 minutes
Supta Vajra Asana	3 minutes
Mayur Asana	2 minutes
Shava Asana	5 minutes

15

Massage Techniques to Slim Body

Massage Therapy

What It Is?

Massage therapy is a technique in which muscles and other soft tissues are pressed, rubbed, and otherwise manipulated. There are several forms of massage, for example is a gentle form of muscular manipulations used primarily for relaxation and stress relief.

How Does It Works?

Pain causes the nervous system to stimulate muscles to contract. The contractions cause more pain, which result in more contractions. Unless the pain-contraction cycle is interrupted, it is hard to find relief. Massage is a way of breaking this cycle. It persuades muscles to relax and lengthen. It brings pain-relieving oxygen and blood to the muscles. And may remove irritating waste materials. In addition, just being touched, it has a deep relaxing and therapeutic effect on the body, although the mechanisms in this effect are not fully understood.

What Can It Do For You?

Massage therapy is effective for any type of pain in body's soft tissues and melt fats and slim down the particular area. This includes back, neck and shoulder pain, headaches caused by tense muscles in the face and scalp besides trimming the whole body.

Is It Safe?

Since massage therapy involves manipulating parts of the body, there is always the possibility that it will make things worse. If you have any type of pain, it is important to see the doctor before turning to massage. Massage should never be done on areas where there is extensive bruising or other kinds of tissue damage. If you are pregnant, have circulatory problems or any unusual condition, get the clearance from your doctor before starting massage therapy. Always let your massage therapist know about your condition, as many are trained to work conservatively in such situations.

Slimming and Massage – The Magic of Hands

The word Massage has been derived from the Arabic word 'Masah' – which means 'the magic of hands'. Massage is one of the easiest way for attaining and maintaining health. Youth, vigor, beauty, slimming, aches and pains, insomnia, tension and stress can be alleviated with a simple instrument-hands. A touch of massage has great value in maintaining beauty, charm and attractive slim body. Experts advise couples to touch each other more often as this can prevent physical and mental illness in a human body. Massage improves circulation, relaxes muscles, aids digestion by stimulating the lymphatic system. It eliminates waste products, provides energy, refreshes and revitalizes the body.

To achieve beneficial results, it is important that the massage is given in a comfortable environment. Choose a warm, peaceful place with dim lights. Always lie on a firm padded surface to relax back and the stomach. Place a cushion under the knees to reduce the arch of the lower back. Also place a folded towel or a small cushion under the head to raise it about an inch or so. A bed may be ideal if you want to give a soothing massage, which can leave you relaxed and sleepy. Keep your back straight throughout the massage and use the weight of your body to give rhythm and depth to the massage. Keep your feet wide apart and bend the knees so that you can lean into the strokes. Never stay in one position for long while massaging. Wear loose-fitting, washable clothes and flat shoes or be bare-footed. Remove all ornaments before giving a massage as it can cause scratches on the skin while giving the massage. When massaging back, put a small cushion or rolled towel under the ankles. A cushion under the waist and one shoulder helps provide relaxing massage.The following exercises keep the hands supple:

1. Hold a rubber ball in one hand and squeeze. Then follow this procedure on the other hand. Relax the fingers repeatedly.
2. Rotate and stretch each finger and thumb in each direction one by one.
3. Press and hold the fingers against each other.

Important Tips for Massage Techniques

1. A rhythmic massage sends waves of relaxation though out the body.
2. If you feel pain or are uncomfortable during the massage, inform the masseur.
3. Mould your hands to the contours of the body.
4. Vary your pressure from vary light to very strong. The massage should be lighter over bony areas and firmer over the muscles.
5. Do not apply heavy pressure when massaging.
6. Concentrate on the massage. Avoid talking when massaging.

7. To give a good massage, be totally relaxed.
8. Do not worry if your initial movements seem clumsy. Practice makes one perfect.

Do Not Massage If You are Suffering From

1. An infection.
2. A contagious disease of the skin.
3. High temperature.
4. Skin infection, bruises or acute inflammation.
5. An inflammatory condition such as thrombosis or phlebitis.
6. Serious inflammatory cases of the joints and in tubercular joints.
7. Suffer from infectious diseases like diphtheria and gonorrhea, which causes formation of pus. The massage may spread the pus to the entire system.

Sprains and bruises can be cured by massage. In these cases, the affected parts should first be bathed with hot water, followed by massage done for few minutes. Gentle stroking and kneading movements are recommended on and around the injured tissues. Muscles constitute one-half of the weight of human body and they are capable of holding half the blood supply. With muscles constituting such a large portion of the body, it becomes all the more important that they are kept nourished. Massage can provide additional nourishment to the muscular tissues.

Nerve compression is recommended for soothing nerves, as a result blood circulation will increase

The Healing Power of Massage

1. *Lymph Drainage*: The lymphatic system acts as a purifying and drainage system and plays an important part in fighting infection and developing immunity. There are lymph vessels and nodes throughout the body. The nodes are present in the neck, armpits, groin, behind the knees and on the inside of the elbows. Massage can energize the lymph throughout the body, thus eliminating waste and strengthening the immune system.

2. *Fight System*: A stressed mind becomes calm, quiet, peaceful and refreshed after a massage. High blood pressure and heart diseases are related to stress. Disorders such as cancer, rheumatism, headaches, backache, acne and pimples, infertility and other infectious skin diseases are more likely to develop when resistance is low. Massage helps to reduce physical as well as emotional stress and relax taut muscles enabling the body and mind to relax.

3. *Insomnia Relief*: In insomnia, general massage during sleep promotes sleep and complete relaxation of the body. Keep all your movements smooth, rhythmic and

hypnotic. Massage back, abdomen and feet using rhythmic stroking movements, which leads to good sleep. There are points when pressed, induce good sleep:

- Press between eyebrows with your thumb holding the pressure for 10 to 15 seconds, then release.

- Press with your thumbs inside of your wrist below your little finger holding pressure for 10 to 15 seconds. Then repeat on other wrist.

- Press the bone of ankle with thumb on inside of your ankle resting your little finger on the bony prominence and the index finger behind the shin bone for ten seconds on each ankle.

4. *Headache and Migraine*: Massage helps in dispelling headaches and migraines. Generally, headaches are caused by changes in blood pressure in blood vessels. Massage relaxes muscle, which allow blood to flow freely, alleviating headache. Cottonseed oil is most commonly used for massaging. But butter is used for filling cheeks, neck and breast enlargement. Oil should not be used by persons have excessive body hair. Such persons should massage with talcum powder. The oil should be washed off completely after the massage.

Do general body massage for 30 to 40 minutes and local body massage for 10 to 15 minutes.

Any area of the body that feels stiff and taut needs extra massage to remove tension, but do not press too hard, slightly increase the pressure of massage and move on to the surrounding area. Massage on the back should be the first area to start, then the feet-which helps to relax whole body. The whole body massage (including face and head) should take about 60 minutes. The massage technique should preferably follow the sequences given below:

1. Right foot and leg, left foot and leg.
2. Left hand and arm, right hand and arm.
3. Abdomen.
4. Back of legs and back.
5. Chest, face and head.

Massage with Aromatic Oils

Massage with essential oils is very useful for the skin, vigor and vitality. Use a light vegetable oil scented with few drops of essential oil for massage. Do not pour the oil directly on to the body. Pour about a teaspoon of oil into the palm, then rub your hands together to warm them slightly and massage. Essential oils blended with massage oil, add new dimension to massage and impart a feeling of luxury to the massage. The perfume in the oil can help to relax or refresh.

Essential oil are extremely concentrated and must be diluted in carrier oil while using them, otherwise they can cause allergies. About 200 kg of rose petal yield a liter of rose oil and 200 of lavender flowers produce about six liters essential oil. The most common carrier oil are almond, soy, grape-seed, avocado, peach and wheat-germ oils (very rich in Vitamin E and acts as an anti-oxidant). To dilute an essential oil, one to three drops are mixed with five teaspoons of carrier oil.

Basic Techniques of Massage

Once you have mastered a few basic massage movements, you can give a complete body massage. The various movements are as under:

1. *Stroking*: The rhythmic flowing movement is very common, in which slow movements applied by the palms and fingertips of both hands side by side leave a calming effect. Brisk movements are, however, stimulating. Apply a steady, even pressure, molding hands to the shape of the body. Stroking improves circulation, relaxes tense muscles and soothes jangled nerves. Fan stroking is the simplest type of stroking movement used on almost all areas of the body. Start with gliding both hands side by side applying steady, even pressure, especially beneficial to shed of extra fat on back and at the waist. Avoid dragging the skin and keep hands relaxed. Circle stroking

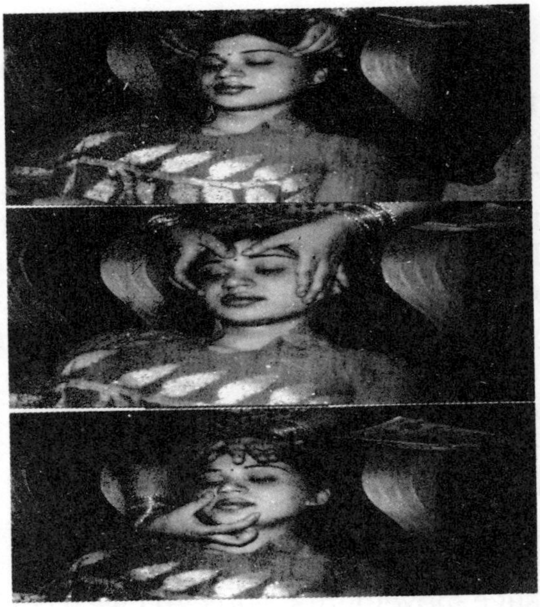

(massage firmly in circles on wide curves), cat stroking (soporific movement slowly), and thumb stroking (applying slight pressure with thumbs) are various stroking movements.

2. *Kneading*: This type of massage is useful on the shoulders and fleshy areas of the body e.g. thighs and hips. It relaxes tense muscles, improves circulation, brings fresh blood and nutrients to the area and eliminates waste products. The movements may be slow and deep or fast and stimulating. Use plenty of oil. Wringing (deeper and more stimulating movement as

if you are wringing out a towel) and light kneading (for less fleshy areas) are various kneading movements.

3. *Pressure*: This movement releases tension in the muscles and is very relaxing when deep, direct pressure is applied. This movement is useful for massaging spine and area around shoulders. Apply pressure gradually and steadily using little oil.

4. *Knuckling*: Useful movement for massaging shoulders, chest, palms and soles. Curl hands into loose fists with the middle section of fingers.

5. *Percussion:* A brisk, bouncy movement usually massaging fleshy, muscular areas. Do not apply this massage movement on bony areas, broken veins and bruises. The movement improves circulation, has calming effect and stimulates the nerves. This massage movement should be applied at the end of massage.

6. *Cradling*: This is a warming up, comforting movement done with both hands relaxed.

7. *Criss-cross Movement*: Glide both hands with fingers facing away and across.

Massage for Slimming Back

Start with stroking movement on the lower and move back towards the head with relaxed hands. Stroke firmly up the back, then pull down on the muscles at the base of neck, across the

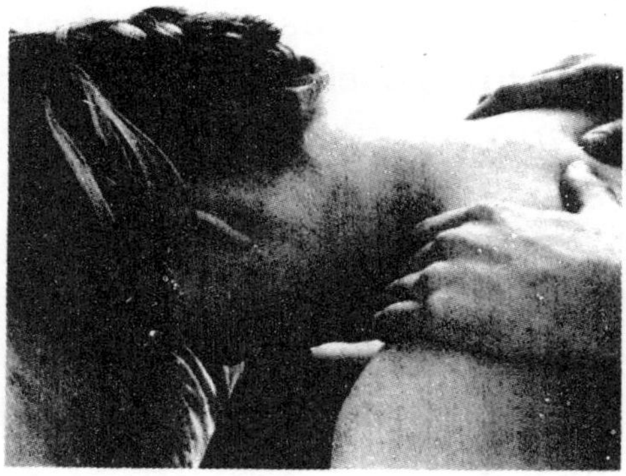

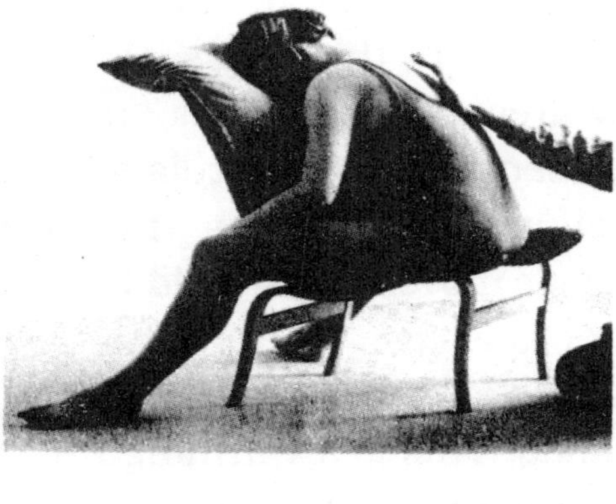

shoulders and upper arms. Other massage movements include Fan Stroking, Pressure Stroking and Kneading.

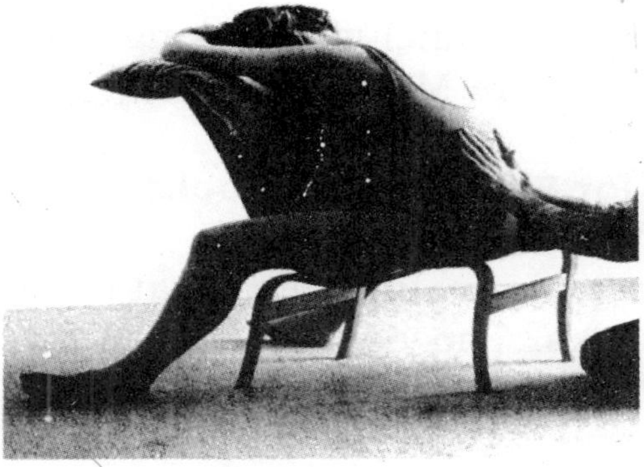

Massage for Slimming Neck and Shoulder

Neck massage is essential as the nerves in this region have to support the weight of the head,

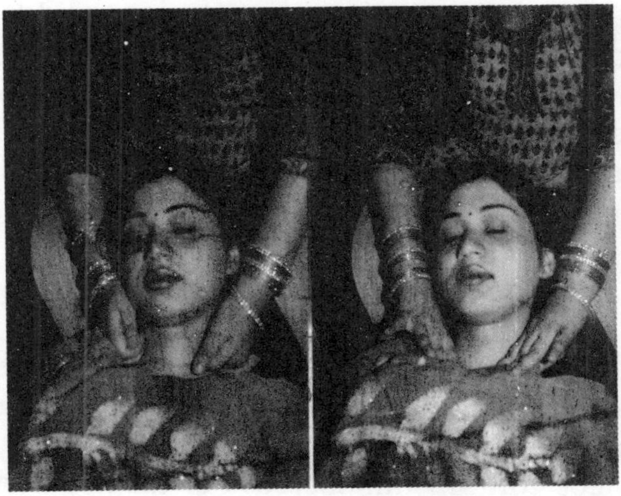

which weighs between five to seven kilograms. The shoulder muscles usually remain tense. Neck and shoulder massage include Stroking, Kneading and Circular Pressure Movements.

Massage for Slimming Buttocks

Tension sometimes exists at the lower back and buttocks. The bottom is usually the most neglected part of the body. Buttock muscles can rid of tension with powerful massage movements such as Circle Stroking, Fan Stroking and Pressure Movements.

Massage for Slimming the Spine

The spine is built of small bones called vertebrae. Between the bones and spongy pads exist discs. Vertebrae mounted on a solid base is attached to the pelvis. Start massage at the neck with index and middle fingers on either side of the spine. Avoid pressing hard on the vertebrae. Stretching movements are deployed for massaging spine.

Leg and Foot Massage Movements

Foot massage not only relaxes thousands thousand of nerve-endings that exist in the sole but also refreshes and stimulates the whole body. The feet contain almost 25% of all the bones in the body. Foot bones and muscles support the weight of the body. For giving foot massage Stroking, Pressure, Rotary Pressure, Passive and Hacking movements are deployed. Legs are built

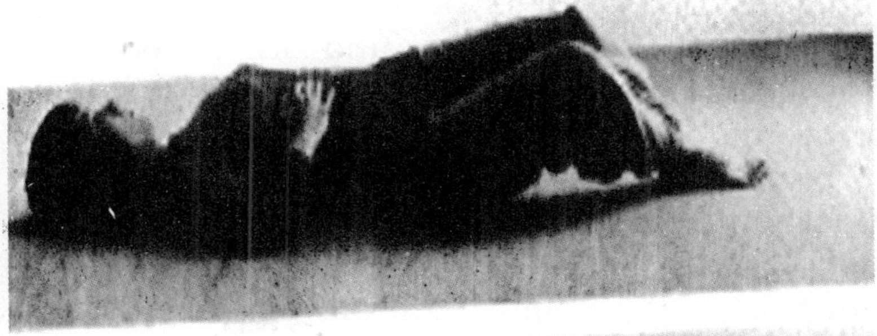

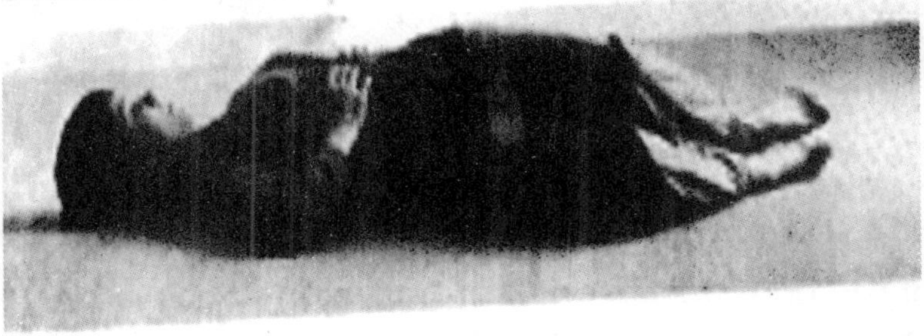

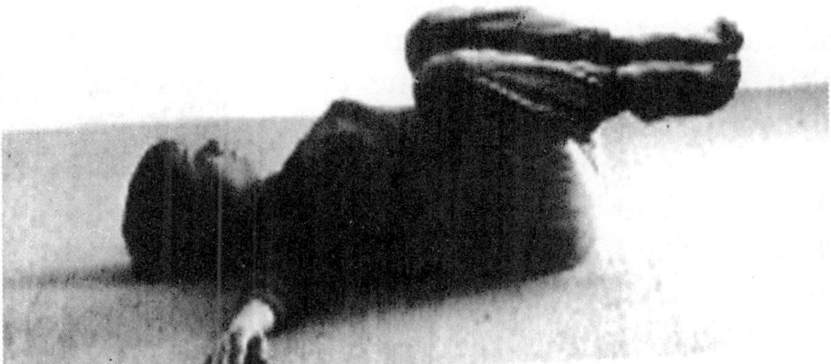

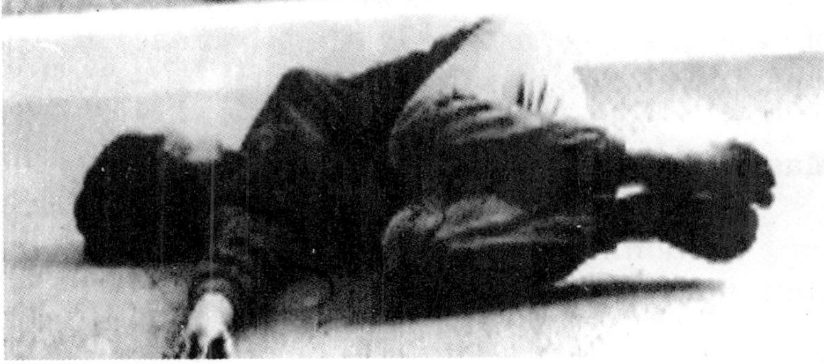

to carry the weight of the body. Legs have strong muscles and bones. Deep, firm massage on muscles will dispel fatigue and bring blood and nutrients to the leg muscles relieving tightness or cramps and prevent varicose veins. Do not forget to press lightly over the bony areas and knees. Massaging legs helps to melt extra fat, reduce puffiness or swelling. Stroking legs and thighs, Kneading calf, Rolling, Thumb circling help to improve the shape of legs, feet and thighs. But do not apply heavy force on the knee joint.

Hand and Arms Massage

Hands are one of the most sensitive parts of the body which contain a large number of nerve endings linked to the brain to register sensation of the whole body. If hands are neglected, the skin of the hands become aged and wrinkled. Hand massage can be given anywhere without inconvenience of getting undressed. The bones of the arms and hands are much more delicate than those of the legs and feet. Tension and tiredness in the arms lead to headache, neck pain and arching shoulders. A regular arms massage alleviates many body disorders. The techniques of hand massage are similar to those used in leg massage.

Massaging Abdomen and Upper Body

Abdominal massage calms the nerves and stimulates the digestive system. Stomach pain is

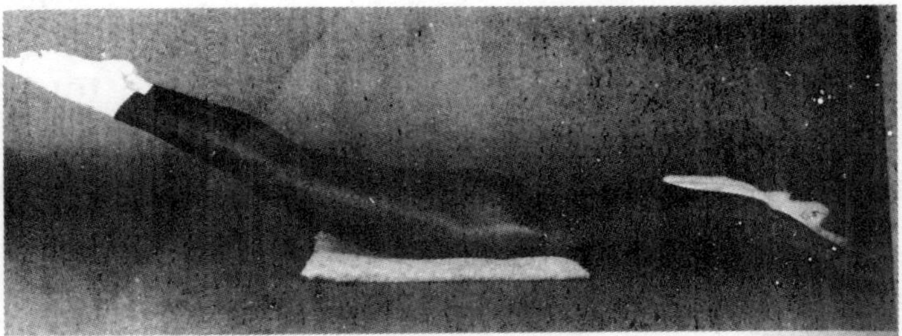

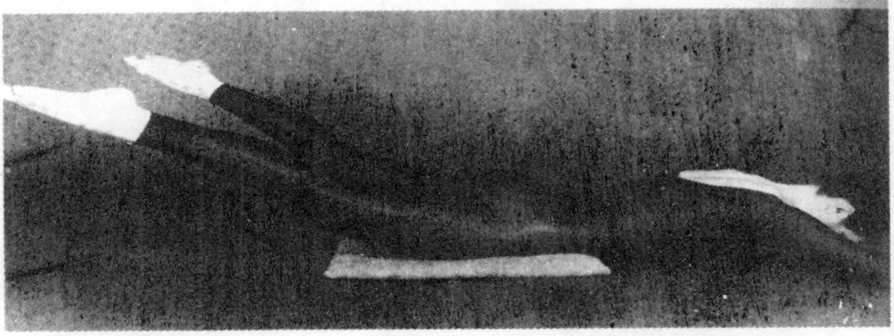

caused by tension, indigestion and bad menstruation. Abdominal massage can soothe them. It relieves constipation, helps in shedding flab and improves skin texture. Pregnant women are not advised a complete abdominal massage. However, a very gentle massage is beneficial for the mother and child in the womb. Massage movements such as Stroking, Circle Stroking and Kneading are recommended for melting fat around abdomen.

Self-massage of Thighs and Abdomen by Pregnant Women

Throughout pregnancy, your body gradually changes shape – you can see your breasts and abdomen swelling. Gentle self-massage not only keeps your skin supple, but also allows you to appreciate your wonderful shape through touch. Self-massage feels good and helps prevent tension during pregnancy developing into pain. If one part of your body is taking too much strain it upsets your overall harmony.

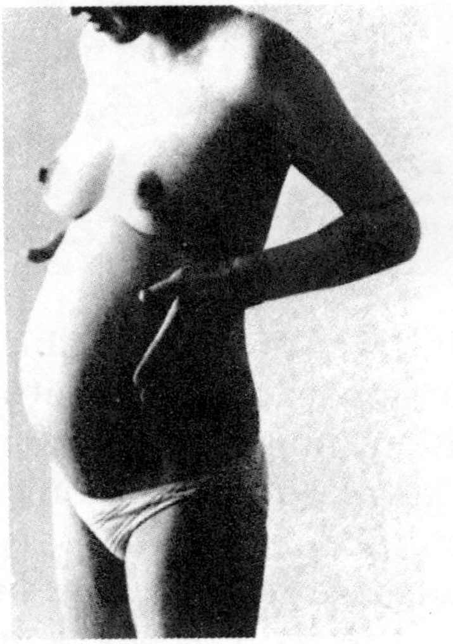

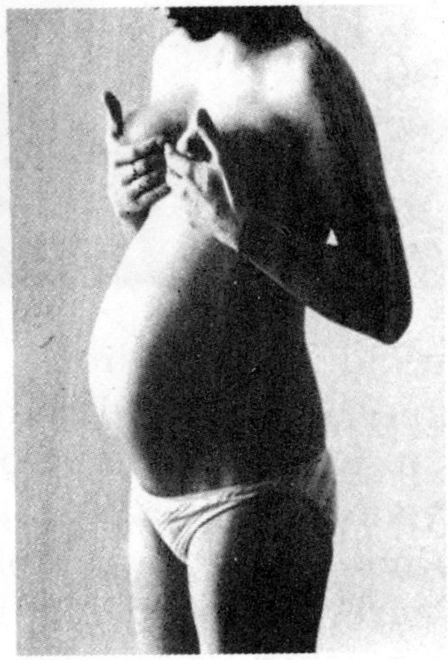

A good time to massage your abdomen, hips, thighs and breasts is after you shower or bathe or when you are getting dressed. Start with your lower abdomen, making slow, gentle, circular strokes with both hands. If you want, try some firmer strokes, going up and over the bulge: imagine that you are lifting the baby back into the pelvis. End the strokes at the top of the bulge and come round and back to the side again. This is particularly comforting towards the end of pregnancy. Start again at the sides, using the same stroke, but continue up and round your breasts.

Massage During Labor Period

Touching, stroking and holding are the most direct ways of communicating with those you love. Within the family, touch and massage not only

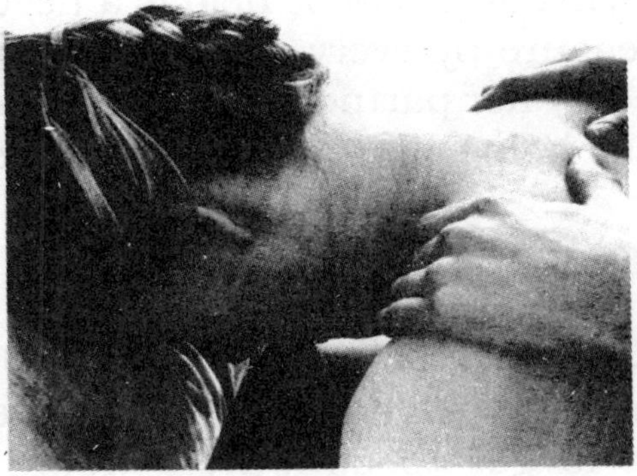

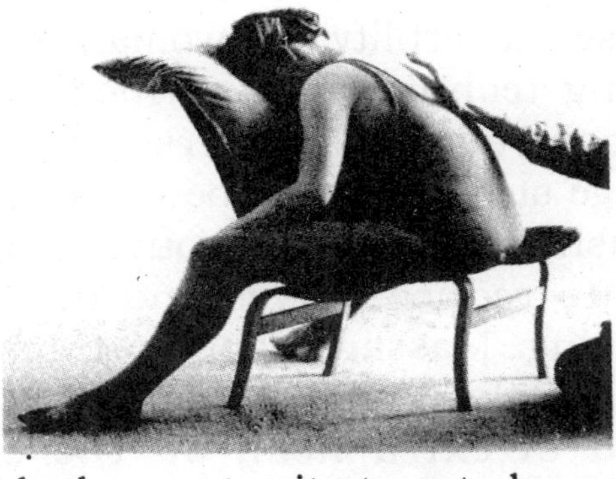

provide an ideal opportunity to get closer to each other, but are the most immediate and effective ways of giving comfort to over-stressed partner during labor. During labor some part of your body may feel uncomfortable, whether from cramps, tension or shivering and you will want massage, stroking or just firm holding to help you feel better. This desire to be held is a need for comfort and pleasure by every woman who prefers being touched by her partner during the stages of labor. This also helps slim the body after delivery.

Massage for Expectant Mothers

Careful, smooth and gentle massage movements benefits woman during pregnancy, but do not forget to consult a doctor. Massage movements help to alleviate many complications such as tension, backache, insomnia and fatty deposits on the body. A pregnant woman should avoid deep pressures and percussion movements. A careful massage during the three trimesters of pregnancy and even before conception helps to increase the fertility of a woman. You can use all stroking techniques described for massaging abdomen, back, shoulders, legs and feet but massage strokes should be gentle and very light. Use cushions under the shoulder, lower back and knees to reduce curves and discomfort while massaging. Massage done by trained masseuse not only makes childbirth easier but also helps to get rid of extra flesh on the body during pregnancy. Lower back and shoulders are areas which help relieve tension while massaging. For back massage, a pregnant woman should lie on her side or sit on a chair (facing towards the back of chair). The various massage movements for a pregnant include:

1. Gentle stroking with one hand, then both hands, one following the other clockwise on the abdomen. Stroking softly on the sides of the waist upward with one hand after the other till both hands reach the navel. Now gently glide the hands towards the abdomen and move down the sides to complete the stroke.

2. Cup your hands over the navel for a few seconds until you feel the heat, then lift your hands slowly.

3. Leg massage is essentially beneficial as it soothes, relaxes and relieves swelling and pain in the legs. Varicose veins and cramps are some of the problems faced by expectant women. The best remedy is to sleep with legs slightly raised above the level of the head. The sleeping posture relieves swelling in the legs by draining the manual lymphatic system. The system drains waste products from the body and helps to cure many skin disorders like acne, eczema and dermatitis.

If the doctor advises restriction on abdominal massage to expectant mothers, they can go for the arm massage, which has a soothing effect on the body. An arm massage can be given to a pregnant woman gently and rhythmically. Backache and morning sickness are the most common complaints during pregnancy, which can be relieved to a great extent with back massage. Avoid deep pressure to the lower back during the first trimester of pregnancy. Stroking movements gently calm the muscles and several complaints by the expectant mother.

Massage After Childbirth

Deep massage to abdomen for 40 days after the delivery energizes the mother, cures body aches, bring the uterus back to its original position and trim the body. To give abdominal massage to a woman after childbirth the following movements should be applied:

1. Stroke the abdomen in all directions. Knead firmly on hips, then gently across the abdomen. Stroke clockwise in large circles on the abdomen. Apply gentle pressure clockwise on the abdomen. Stroke slowly up the abdomen, starting at the pubic bone and pressing with the heel of your hands.

2. Stroke slowly on the lower abdomen, starting from the pubic bone to the navel. Cup your hands over the navel and hold for few minutes until you feel heat accumulating under the hands. Then lift hand slowly.

16

Periods, Pregnancy and Post-natal Fitness Tips

Correct Sitting Position While Sitting on a Chair

- Starting Position: Sit on a hard chair or stool.
- Feet: Ensure that the feet are resting on the floor, hip-width apart and pointing very slightly outwards.
- Knees: Are bent comfortably, at about a right angle.
- Thighs: The thighs are hip-width apart.
- Pelvis: Control the tilt of the pelvis, as in standing.
- Ribs: Lift the rib cage up away from the hips by stretching your upper back, so there is length in the center of the body. Do not keep the abdomen pulled in tightly.
- Shoulder: The shoulders are down away from the ears.

- The back of the neck is lengthened upwards.
- Head: The chin is held at about a right angle to the front of the neck, ears directly above the shoulders.

Exercises sitting on a chair

How to Get Rid of a Double Chin?

Neck exercise programme starts off by stretching and strengthening the muscles of the neck, shoulder and the chin. It is very important to work on these areas first because any tendency, tenseness and tightness there will increase as you work other areas of the body. The neck and shoulders always have priority, so if you find you are straining them in order to do something in another part of the body, beware. The exercise probably will not do you good. The following exercise movements should be performed:

1. Head tilting forward, which stretch and strengthen the straight muscles of the neck and upper back. Carefully tilt the head forward, keeping the chin in, until you feel a stretch in the back of the neck. Lift the head a little if the stretch becomes too much. Now tilt the head forward until you feel muscles stretched. Repeat three to four times.

2. Head pressing backwards, which strengthens the muscles at the back of the

neck by static muscle work. Never overdo neck work. If you find this exercise difficult, try it lying on the floor, so the head is supported, and press the head into the floor.

3. Head tilting sideways, which stretches and strengthens the muscles at the sides of the neck. Do not repeat side stretching of the neck more than once on each side.

4. Head tilting diagonally forwards, which stretches and strengthens the diagonal muscles of the neck and upper back.

Simple Shoulder-blade Squeeze to Melt Extra Fat

This exercise strengthens the muscles, which pull the shoulder blades together and pull

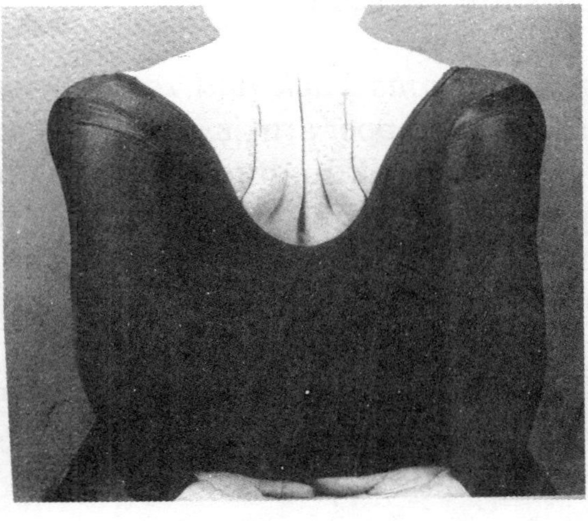

back the arms. This exercise at the same time lifts the ribcage so that it is in better position for the movement of the lower ribs in breathing. To practice this exercise, sit correctly on a chair or stool. Clasp hands loosely behind the back with elbows slightly bent. Draw the shoulder blades together (as shown in the illustration) and at the same time, the upper arms towards each other across the back. Do not straighten the elbows. Rest, keeping the hands in position. Repeat exercise three times in the beginning and gradually increase to six times a day. Do not arch the back.

Arm, Breast and Hands Exercises

These help prevent stiffness in the shoulders, elbow, wrists and finger joints. They also tighten up the contours of the arms, and help to lift loose, saggy breasts. The following exercise movements are suggested:

1. *Pressing arms back and rotation inwards*: Back of the upper arm is a part that so many women complain has 'gone to flab' To tighten up the muscles, encourage inward rotation of the lower arms and shoulder joints, which strengthens muscles across the back. Do not be surprised if the backs of the upper arms feel a little stiff for a day or two after you have done the exercise. It is strong but very effective.

2. *Rotating the arms outwards and inwards*: The rotation of the shoulder joints and lower arms prevent stiffness. In this exercise, lift the elbows slightly and turn the hands outwards fully, straightening the elbows. Repeat this movement as often as you can, Make sure, the rotation in the forearms and shoulder joints should be in a flowing movement. Remember, to keep the shoulders down away from the ears.

3. *Advance rotation of arms*: This movement strengthens the muscles in the shoulder joints that rotate the arms. Raise the lower arms to form right angles at the elbows, keeping the upper arms at shoulder level on both side of the face. Repeat the movement as often as you like. Keep the shoulders down away from the ears.

4. *Breast lifting exercise*: Strengthens the muscles, which lie behind the breasts and help to support it. Breasts start getting swollen during pregnancy, it loose shape and become heavy during lactation period. Rotating the arms in circle strengthen loose muscles. This exercise should be followed by massage with olive oil or a breast massage cream readily available in the market.

5. *Hand stretching exercise*: Stretch the fingers and thumbs to prevent stiffness. Sit on a chair or stool, placing hands on the thighs and palms down. Lift the hands up and stretch out. Open fingers and thumbs as much as possible. Let the hands drop back onto the thighs. Repeat several times. Keep the wrists resting on your thighs and do not lift the shoulders.

Abdominal and Back Exercises

The movements given below help to shorten and tighten up the abdominal muscles in all directions:

1. *Waist side bends*: This exercise movement stretches and strengthens the muscles at the side of the trunk, back and front. It mobilizes the five joints of the lower back. Clasp the hands just above the head, elbows out sideways. Do a three-point pull, Bend sideways to the right as far as you can, keeping the pelvis firmly on the chair. Hold the position for few seconds. Return to initial standing position and repeat on other side. Do not allow the chest to sag or rotate. This exercise tones up abdominal and back muscles, and slim the waist.

2. *Waist twist*: Tones up and mobilizes the diagonal muscles and joints of the abdomen, upper back and the neck. Place hands flat on the upper chest. Twist round to the, turning your head as far as you can. The pelvis must remain facing forwards. Go on pressing round in small further movements, with the head and upper body. Face front again and repeat to the other side. Try not to lift the shoulders.

3. *Waist diagonal bend*: It mobilizes the whole spine, tones up abdominal and back muscles. Sit on a chair or a stool. Clasp hands just above the head, elbows out sideways. Twist to the left as far as you can. Return to starting position, then repeat on right side. Do this exercise three to four times. Do not attempt this exercise if you have any weakness or pain in the lower back.

4. *The pelvic tilt*: Sit on a chair near the front of the seat, hands holding the back. Start rolling the pelvis so that the pubic bone comes up. Straighten the curve of the lower back so that the tummy is compressed. Return to the starting position after 10-15 counts. This exercise helps easy movement of pelvis and mobilizes hip joints and lower back. Keep upright from the waist while doing exercise.

Leg and Feet Exercises

Tired and fleshy feet tend to make you feel tired all over. Foot exercises become pleasant and can be done any time anywhere whenever you have a moment to spare. There are several types of exercises for the feet:

1. *Ankle and foot joint exercise*: This exercise strengthen, mobilize the ankles and joints of the feet. Sit comfortably on a chair. Place the feet slightly forwards. Keep heels on the

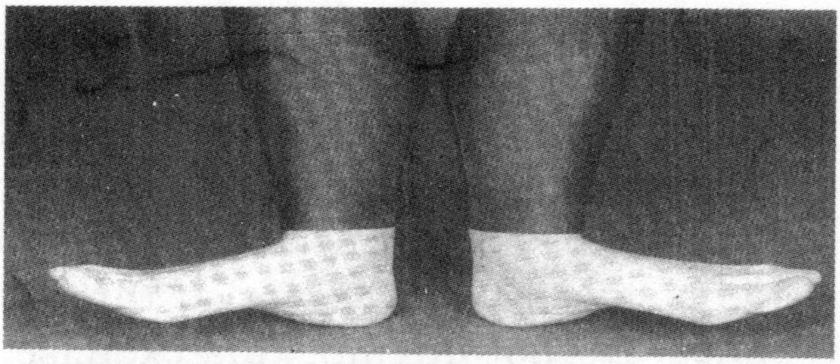

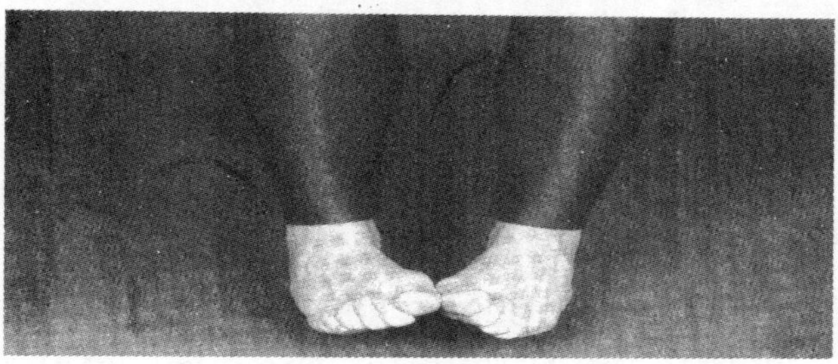

floor and knees together throughout the exercise. Brush the feet outwards along the floor lifting and turning them as much as possible so that the big toes point towards the outside of the calves. Now drop the feet and brush them inwards along the floor lifting and turning them as much as possible so that the big toes point towards the inside of the calves.

2. Another Instep exercise to strengthen the small muscles of the feet that support the arches can be performed by drawing the

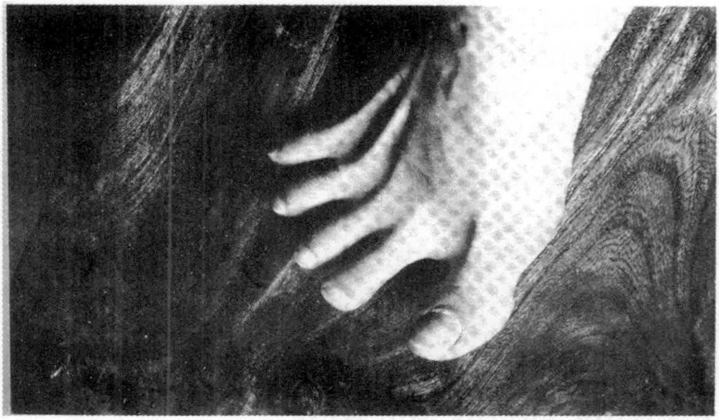

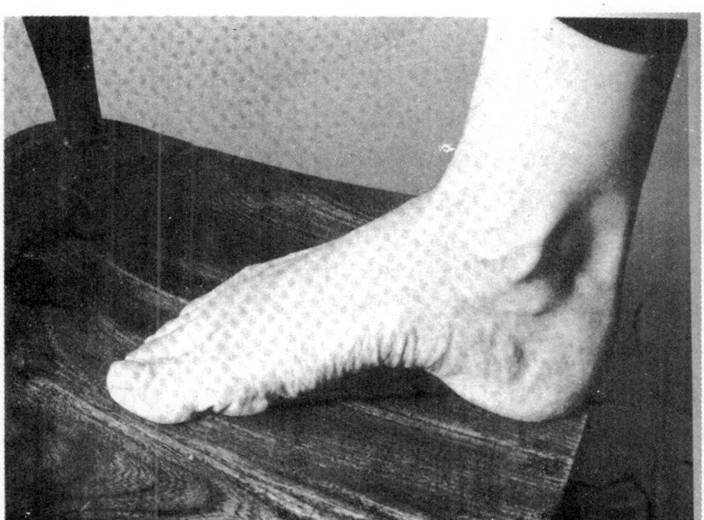

toes straight towards the heel sliding along the floor, so that you hump up the joints where the toes attach to the feet. Now slide the toes out along the floor and stretch them trying to open out the toes.

Buttock Exercises

Tightening the buttocks make childbirth easier and painless. This exercise is particularly applicable to women who usually have more fat around the buttocks than men. Sit correctly on chair or a stool. Move the feet slightly forwards, hands resting on the upper chest. Then do a pelvic tilt pressing the thighs downwards and rotating them outwards. Repeat several times and stop when you feel uncomfortable.

Exercising Thighs and Hips

Tighten the front of thighs that increases the circulation in the muscles of thighs and hips. Sit on a chair or a stool with hand on hips. Do a pelvic tilt and turn the thighs outwards. Left feet should remain on the ground during exercise, whereas lift right leg off the floor, knees slightly bent and feet bent upwards. Now straighten the right leg quickly and start kicks, pushing the heel away from you. Repeat the kick several times until the leg begins to tire. Return to the starting position and repeat exercise with the other leg. If you have painful knees, leave out this exercise or gently bend and stretch the leg instead of kicking.

Exercises Lying on the Floor

These types of exercises performed on the floor are recommended to women during periods and pregnancy. You can allow your body, through neglect to sag, bulge and spread. It also gives a brief introduction to the technique of physiological relaxation and adds grace and vigor to the body.

Exercises to Strengthen the Muscles of Back

Sit on the floor with legs bent, knees dropped outwards and the soles of the feet together. Clasp hands around the toes and press soles of both feet. If you are feeling uncomfortable, put a cushion under your bottom and hold the ankles instead of the toes. Press the knees towards the floor. Straighten the back, lifting the chest. This exercise leaves the following effects:

- Strengthens the back muscles.
- Mobilizes the hip joints.
- Stretches the Inward Rotators and Abductors of the hips.

Exercises to Stretch Thigh Muscles

Sit on the floor with the legs as far apart and straight as reasonably comfortable. Knees caps should face upwards. Loosely fist the hands and press them on the floor behind. This posture strengthens the back muscles, mobilizes the hip joints and stretches inside thigh muscles.

To stretch the muscles on the back of thighs and back of lower legs, sit on the floor with legs spread straight forwards, feet together pointing upwards towards the face. Loosely fist the hands and press them on the floor behind. Put a cushion under your bottom and bend your knees a little if you find this position difficult. This exercise also helps to strengthen back muscles and mobilize the hip joints.

Back Control Muscle Exercise

Sit on the floor with legs spread straight forward. Place a towel around the middle of the feet and hold it in both hands. Pull the towel and lower the trunk slowly forwards, keeping back to remain straight and the chest lifted. Hold the position for at least 30 seconds. Repeat this exercise for few times. Inhale as you lift trunk, exhale as you lower the trunk. Finally lower the trunk and clasp the hands under the feet to relax. Pregnant women should do this exercise without any pressure.

Pelvic Exercise

Lie on the floor straight. Bend the knees up, keeping feet flat on the floor, hip-width apart. Roll the pelvis so that the pubic bone in front comes up towards your nose. Your lower back will press onto the floor and your tummy will be compressed. Let the pelvis roll back to the starting position. Repeat as often as you can do uncomfortably. Breath in when starting the position, breath out as you tilt the pelvis upwards and breathe normally as you hold the position. Breath in as the pelvis rolls back to starting position. Keep the shoulders down away from the ears and the top half of the body quite at ease.

For mobilizing the joints of the lumbar region (lower back), tighten muscles at the sides of the waist. Do not lift the hips off the floor as you work. Only move the legs as a result of the action by the pelvis. This exercise is particularly helpful for those who tend to get stiff in the lower back, especially after sleep. This exercise can also be done in standing and lifting the pelvis. The exercise is very useful if you have to stand for long periods.

Leg-raising Exercise for Thighs and Buttocks

Posture-1: Lie on your right side with the body and legs in a straight line. Keeping both knees

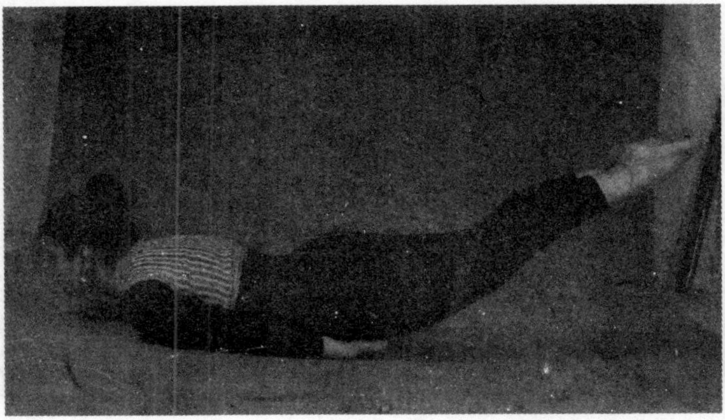

facing forwards, lift left leg up until the pelvis begins to lift sideway. Hold the position for ten seconds. Lower the leg slowly and let the leg rest on the floor. Hold for ten seconds and repeat as often as you can do comfortably. Now roll over and repeat the sequence on the other side.

Posture-2: Lie on your right side. Lift the left leg up to about ten inches off the floor at an angle 45 degrees. Swing lifted leg back and turn it out allowing the chest and pelvis to come forward a little. Lower the leg to the floor. Now repeat the sequence on the other side. This exercise can also be done standing. Do not arch or hollow the back.

Leg-raising Exercise for Toning the Loose Muscles of Buttocks and Thighs

Women during periods, pregnancy and soon after childbirth should avoid this exercise.

Posture-1: To do this exercise, lie on the tummy with a cushion under the pelvis. Bend the elbows

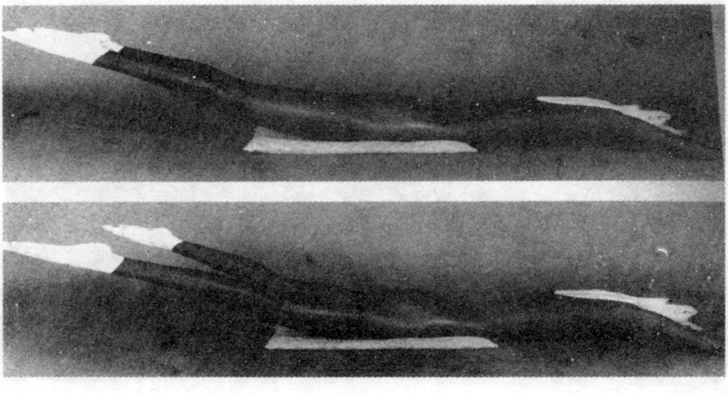

and put the hands in front of you on the floor. Rest your forehead on the hands. Now raise both legs, trying to lift the thighs off the floor. Hold the position for a few moments, and lower the legs gently to the floor.

Position-2: Perform this exercise as in case of Posture-1 except taking the legs apart. Make small circles clockwise, then anti-clockwise with the legs at the hip joints. Breathe Normal do not hold the breath. If your legs are weak, lift only one leg at a time. If this exercise hurts your back, do not perform it. This exercise is not suitable for pregnant women.

Stretching the Muscles of the Back and Neck

1. Kneel on the ground. Rest your bottom on or near the heel.

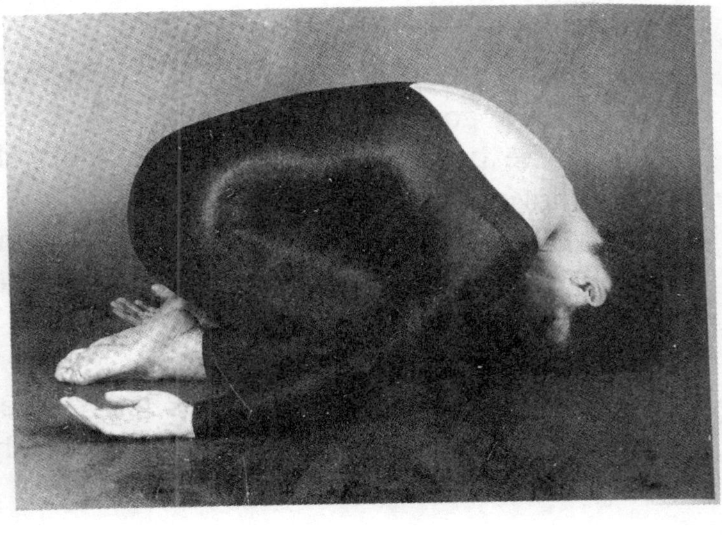

2. Curl forwards and tuck your head in towards your knees.
3. Pull your shoulders down and rest the hands, palms up, on the floor on sides.
4. Rest in this position for as long as you like.

Correct Standing Position

Hold the body in balance for standing and walking.

1. *Feet*: Stand with the feet hip-width apart and very slightly turned out with the weight evenly distributed between the balls of the feet and the heels.
2. *Knees*: The knees are at ease so they neither pull back tightly nor bend forwards.
3. *Pelvis*: Control the tilt of the pelvis so that it is not dropped too far down in front or lifted too far up.
4. *Ribs*: The ribcage is slightly lifted so that there is a good space between it and the hips. The upper back of the body controls this movement.
5. *Shoulders*: The shoulders are down, away from the ears. When viewed from the side, they should be directly above the ankles.
6. *Arms*: Hang freely at the sides.
7. *Neck*: The back of the neck is lengthened upwards so that the chin is at about a right angle to the front of the neck.

8. *Head*: Feel you are lifting the crown of the head upwards. Ears directly above the shoulders.

DETOX – To Eliminate Toxins and Get Rid of Extra Fat

Daily care can help keep your whole body smooth and soft. But during periods, pregnancy and after delivering of child, many times specific problems, usually accumulation of flesh on various parts of the body, arise which need particular attention. **DETOX** is the best way to eliminate toxins, get radiant skin and get rid of extra fat.

Easy Ways to Give Your Body Detox for Slimming

You need a beauty detox if:

- If you are overweight.
- Fat has accumulated on visible parts of your body and breasts.
- You have cellulite.
- The skin looks bumpy on upper arms.
- Your body feels no energy and you have poor circulation.
- Your skin on the face and body is very dry and looks chalky.
- Your skin looks gray and lifeless.
- You have dark circles and puffiness around the eyes.

- You are getting breakouts on the face and body.

The following are easy ways to give detox to beautify and slim down:

Massage

It leaves a miraculous effect to improve circulation and lymph drainage to banish cellulite.

Aroma Treatment

Massaging fatty parts of the body with Aroma oils, mixing up about five drops of pure essential oil (such as lemon, juniper) with 10 ml of a carrier oil (preferably sweet almond oil) is very useful to melt fat. Massage as long as it takes the oil to be absorbed on the areas of body such as your hips, butt, thigh and abdomen once a day.

Spa Massage

It helps a good circulation if applied after a bath while the skin is still damp and warm. Mix to the massage oil a body contouring cream (readily available in the market) for better and smoothing results.

Body Brush

It is excellent treatment for busting cellulite, which smoothes and firms the skin. Do not neglect your back. Brush your back, legs and arms towards your heart in a circular, clockwise movement through your tummy (which is worst affected with extra flesh and wrinkles after childbirth).

Face and Body Masking

Masking is a good flush out and helps to clear a congested skin using stimulating herbal ingredients such as rosemary and eucalyptus, which leave dehydrating effect on dry as well as oily skins. Mask your skin for 5 to 20 minutes depending upon the condition of wet packs, which help to lower high temperature, raise a subnormal temperature, relieve inner congestion, promote elimination, stimulates sluggish circulation – all these help to shed-off extra fat.

Steam Bath

Also known as Sauna Bath, is one of the most important water treatment which induces perspiration. Sauna helps losing a couple of kilos, but you will put them again if eat or drink immediately after having bath. Do not drink anything for at least one hour after the bath. Steam bath (sauna) along with exercise and good diet can do wonders in reducing weight. To exercise 15 minutes in sauna is equivalent to running two kilometers. Toxins are eliminated through the skin in sauna bath, which helps

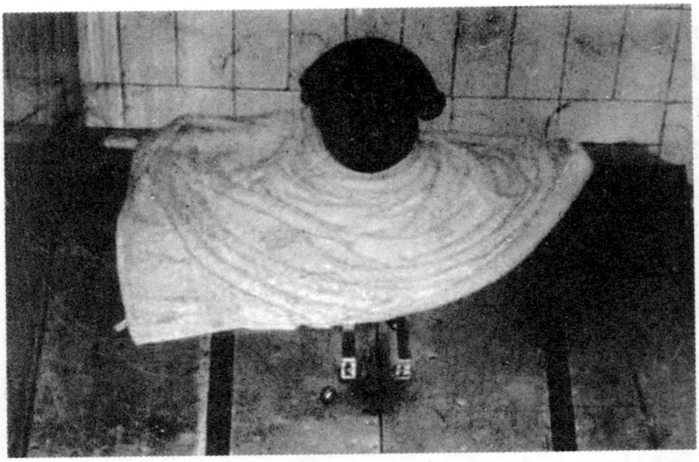

clearing cellulite besides curing many skin problems like acne, dull and lifeless complexion.

Hip Baths

An hip bath is one of the most useful forms of hydrotherapy, in which a bath is taken in a tub filled with water which involves only the hips and

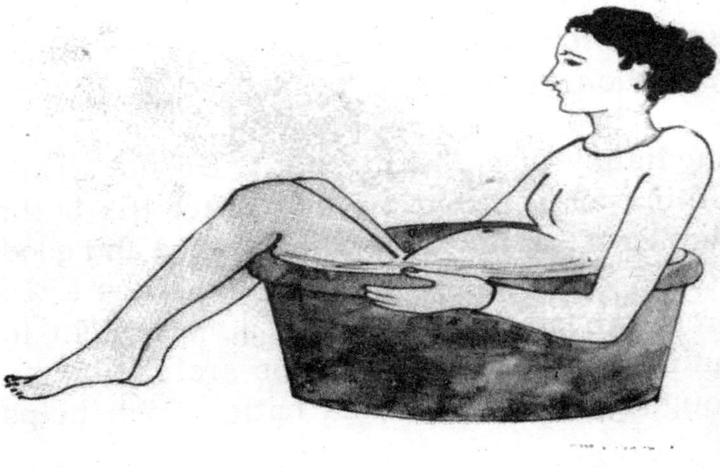

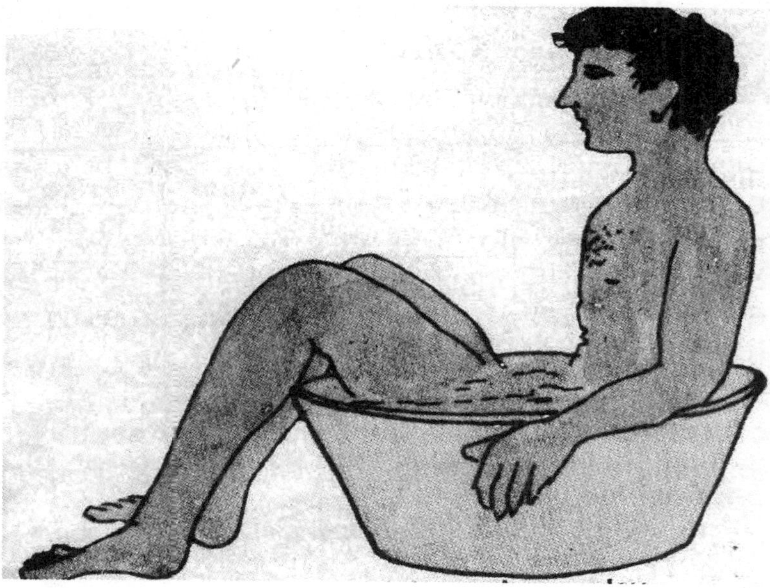

the abdominal region. The water level in the tub covers the hips up to the navel when the patient sits in it. Hip bath is taken in cold, hot, neutral water having alternate temperature. Rub the abdomen briskly from navel downwards and across the body with a coarse wet cloth for excellent results in eliminating obesity. Such baths help to reduce extra flesh from the hips and abdomen.

Cold Hip Bath is taken for 30 minutes in water having temperature varying between 10-18 degree C.

Hot Hip Bath is taken for eight to ten minutes at water temperature 40 to 45 degree C. Do not apply friction to the abdomen in this bath.

Hot and Cold Hip Bath is a treatment in which the patient sits in the hot tub (water temperature 40-45 degree C) for five minutes, followed by a cold bath (water temperature 10-18 degree C) for three minutes. This bath relieves chronic inflammatory conditions of the pelvic and cellulite. These hip baths are very useful in fighting obesity, relieve constipation, indigestion, diarrhea, dysentery and cure uterine problems such as irregular menstruation, uterine infection, pelvic inflammation, piles, hepatic congestion, congestion of prostate glands, seminal weakness, impotency, sterility, ovarian displacement, dilation of stomach and colon, hemorrhage of the bladder and many other problems which effect beauty and body.

Lymphatic Drainage Therapy

This therapy needs gentle pressure on the lymphatic system to move waste materials out of the body quickly. These waste materials are drained out through urine and relieve cellulite.

Sandalwood Treatment

It is best suited for water retention, is diuretic and diaphoretic and leads to detoxification. Cellulite triggers skin to sweat and release toxins, and act as disinfectant. Sandalwood unlocks trapped fluid and toxins been stored in the tissues, which helps reduce fatness in the body.

Panchkarma Massage

Panchkarma means '5 action', which is an ancient scientific system for detoxification and rejuvenate the whole body system. It relieves stress on the muscles and internal organs, balances body, mind and soul. Vigorous and gentle rhythmic soothing movements applied on the body help to achieve maximum results in burning fat.

Shiatsu Therapy

This therapy is also known as acupressure. There are nearly 600 Shiatsu Points on the human body. Pressure on these points with both hands moving rhythmically along the meridians from one point to the other, pressing each from three to seven seconds, produce energy that flows in the body and improve the circulation and induce relaxation. Shiatsu therapy is a wide subject, but here only a couple of tips are being given, which help to reduce fat.

1. When pressing on front abdominal area, at one inch either side of the navel, reduces fat accumulated in the belly area, besides stimulating and energizing the muscles of abdomen.

2. When pressing on the front abdominal area, at three inches below the navel, helps weight reduction and cures cellulite.

Surya Mudra

This 'mudra' helps in reducing body fat. Bend the ring finger and press it with the tip of thumb for 10 to 15 minutes daily in the morning and in the evening. Perform this mudra preferably sitting in Yoga posture - *Padma Asana*.

17

And Don't Neglect Your Body and Diet

Areas of Special Care

Daily care can help you keep your whole body smooth and soft. But sometime specific problems arise which need particular attention. Here are details about improving your body, skin texture, color and tone.

Neck

This can be one of the most neglected areas of the body, yet it is neck which gives away a woman's age almost before anything else. Include it in all beauty routines-cleansing, toning and nourishing. If your neck is crepey — looking and covered in fine lines, use a special nourishing cream every night before going to bed and stimulate circulation with gentle massage, moving your hands alternately from the base of the throat upwards to the chin in a flowing movement. Stroking, kneading and circular pressure massage movements are applied to have comfort, ease mental tension and dissolve fat.

Upper Arms

If faulty circulation makes your arms look mottled and unattractive. Rub them briskly with a friction mitt when you are in the bath and then rinse with hot and cold water alternatively. Add a little Epsom salt in bath water. Beware of sitting with your arms uncovered in the sun or too close to an open fire and of sudden changes in temperature. If your upper arms are thick, with a tough-looking skin, which looks like pale orange peel, it may be affected by cellulite. This condition, usually found on the thighs, stomach and on the upper arms, is caused by an infection of the subcutaneous skin tissues. Very stringent massage can help to break up the deposits of fat. A diet, which includes plenty of fresh fruit (particularly orange and lemon) and green vegetables can help too. Try a professional massage.

Elbows

Take a look at your elbows. If they are dry, wrinkled and red-looking, give them a beauty treatment every day. Soften elbows and make them whiter by leaning them in halves of fresh lemon. If the elbows are very sore, apply a soothing paste made from a cup of oatmeal mixed with a little boiling milk. Allow this to cool smooth it on your elbows and leave it there for few minutes, then wash it off with lukewarm water.

Stomach

Stretch marks and fat on stomach (usually after childbirth) result when the fibers beneath the surface of the skin weaken and the normal, elasticity of the skin is not enough. The marks and extra flesh most commonly occur just after childbirth, but they can also appear suddenly in puberty when the growth rate is very fast. The application of olive or baby oil throughout the period of pregnancy and immediately after the birth of the baby is essential. However, if the marks have appeared, lubricating the skin can certainly help to minimize the less severe one. The marks and the extra deposits of fat on the body may disappear with the regular application of a cream containing a large concentration of vitamin E or by massaging the body. Most serious stretch marks are, however, difficult to disguise and sometimes surgery may be recommended.

Breasts and Abdomen

If you have mottled-looking skin on the breasts or the breasts have sag or are extra heavy, stimulate circulation with alternative rinses of hot and cold water. It will help to minimize the problem and make your bosom firmer. If the skin looks

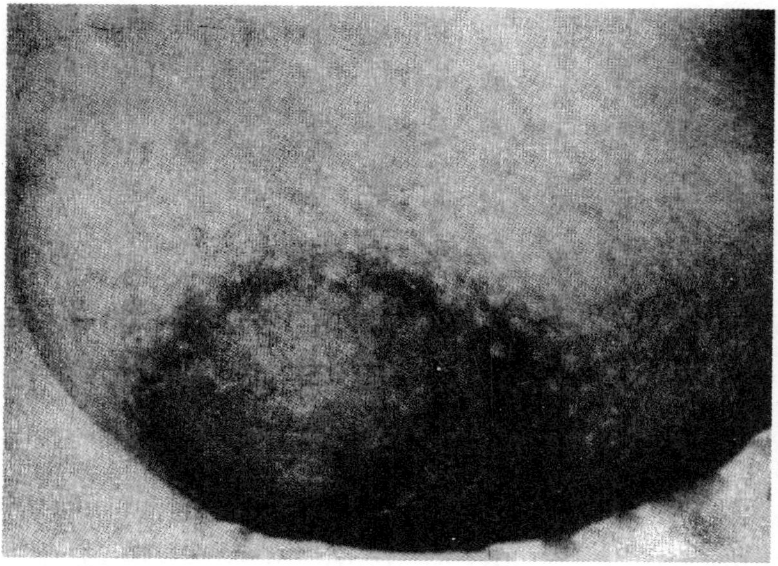

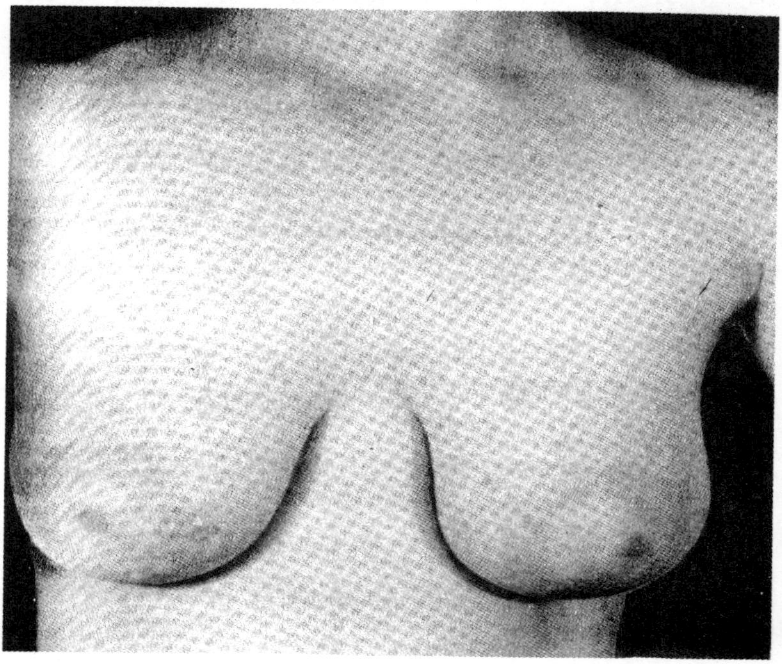

wrinkled and sagging after the childbirth or breast-feeding, use a good moisturizing cream and follow the exercise to keep breast fit. A good time to massage your abdomen, hips, thighs and breasts is after your shower or bathe or when you are getting dressed. Start with your lower abdomen, making slow, gentle, circular strokes with both hands. Then, if you want, try some firm strokes, going up and over the bulge, imagining that you are lifting the baby back into the pelvis. End the strokes at the top of the bulge and come round and back to the side again. This is particularly comforting towards the end of pregnancy. Start again at the sides, using the same strokes, but continue up and round your breasts. Stroking, circle stroking, rotary pressure movement, kneading and feather stroking are important massage movements applied to shed off extra weight.

Thighs, Knees and Bottom

The 'orange peel' skin here is usually caused by cellulite and needs tough, regular massage by an expert massager. Mottled skin on the thighs indicates faulty circulation and you can improve this with the help of a friction mitt used in circular motion. Rough, red and fleshy knees respond to pampering with body lotion and nourishing moisturizing cream. Rub them with baby oil or olive oil after bathing.

Bottoms are sun and air-starved. Even in summer, they are kept covered, so no wonder they tend to look pale and pasty. Nude sunbathing is impractical for most of men and women, but instead of that you can use a ultra-violet lamp for few seconds everyday or have a course of ultra-violet treatments. This will also help melting extra fat deposits. Always moisturize this area of your body with plenty of body lotion. If the flesh is bulgy and bumpy, literally pummel it into shape by bumping each cheek against a wall for a count of 10 everyday. Pinching the flesh on your bottom when you are in the bath is also good for circulation and shape. Walking provides good bottom-shaping exercise, and walking on your bottom will help to reduce bulges and tone the skin.

Back

Spotty backs are often a problem for people who tend to have greasy skin. The over-active sebaceous glands cause the greasy secretions. Spots are themselves stimulated by hormonal activity in the body, particularly in adolescence. The only remedy is to keep the skin scrupulously clean by washing with a medicated liquid soap daily. To avoid unnecessary irritation, choose cotton for the vest, bra, blouse or T-shirt. Apply a medicated cleansing lotion and anti-acne cream to dry up the excess grease at bedtime. If a spot appears on your back just before you plan to wear a low-backed or backless dress, disguise it with a medicated made-up stick matching to your skin-tone.

Here are few tips for the skin:

1. Cleansing or rubbing the back is not easy which results in accumulation of layers of dirt on the back. Women with oily skin suffer a dark patchy skin and rashes. This part becomes itchy and when scratched irritation increases and rashes spread leaving permanent marks. Use medicated soap to heal rashes on the back.
2. Massage the back with mustard oil before taking bath.
3. Rub in some acne lotion at night and wear loose dresses to avoid itching.
4. Rub the back with a paste of 'maida' mixed to un-boiled milk. Leave the paste for ten minutes, then wash it off with cold water.
5. Rubbing lemon is effective for a dark complexioned back.
6. Cut the lemon in two pieces, rub on the back, let the juice dry for ten minutes and wash off with cold water.
7. Unwanted hair on the back, can be hidden by bleaching.
8. Use of face pack on the back ensures a beautiful, soft, lustrous skin. Try a pack of gram-flour mixed with rose water and un-boiled milk. For better results, mix to it few drops of hydrogen per-oxide and mustard

oil. Rub it on the neck and back, let it dry, then wash off. It has a magic effect to clear the skin.

In case of fat deposits on the shoulders and back, massage will help a lot. Stroking, fan stroking and kneading movements from the base of neck, shoulders till hands reach the waist will not only clear fat deposits, but strengthen the spinal cord.

How to do Traditional Thai Massage?

Traditional Thai Massage with complete movements and stretch of every body muscle is a unique combination of acupressure, breathing techniques, gentle stretches and healthy posture. This massage technique stimulates the flow of energy and balance restored to the body – physically, emotionally, mentally and spiritually. Thai massage ensures the following benefits:

1. Promotes circulation of blood and lymph, thus melts excess fat on the body.
2. Release strength and increases energy.
3. Increases flexibility and range of motion.
4. Provides deep relaxation pressure on feet and legs are sedating.
5. Releases point of tension in the body, which blocks the natural flow of energy.
6. Helps hormone stasis balance and harmony.
7. Strengthens the internal organs.

8. Improve blood circulation.
9. Expels out harmful toxins from the body.
10. Promotes inner peace and quite mind.
11. Assists alignment and postural integrity of the body.
12. Most suitable for post-natal mothers.
13. Improves neurological functions.
14. Treats muscular and general relaxation.
15. Helps stress reduction.
16. Relieves body pain and recovery from injury.
17. Restores metabolic balance.

Nutrition Value of Food Products

- Most fruits, particularly citrus fruits, are rich in vitamin C and the sugar in fruits are an instant and natural source of energy.

- Whole-meal grains provide roughage, essential for the digestive system and are a valuable source of vitamins B, E and K, as well as minerals.

- Green leafy vegetables such as cabbage provide vitamin A, B, C and K as well as iron, iodine and other valuable minerals.

- Colorful vegetables are an important source of vitamin A and vitamin C.

- Most vegetable oils are polyunsaturated fats, unlike animal

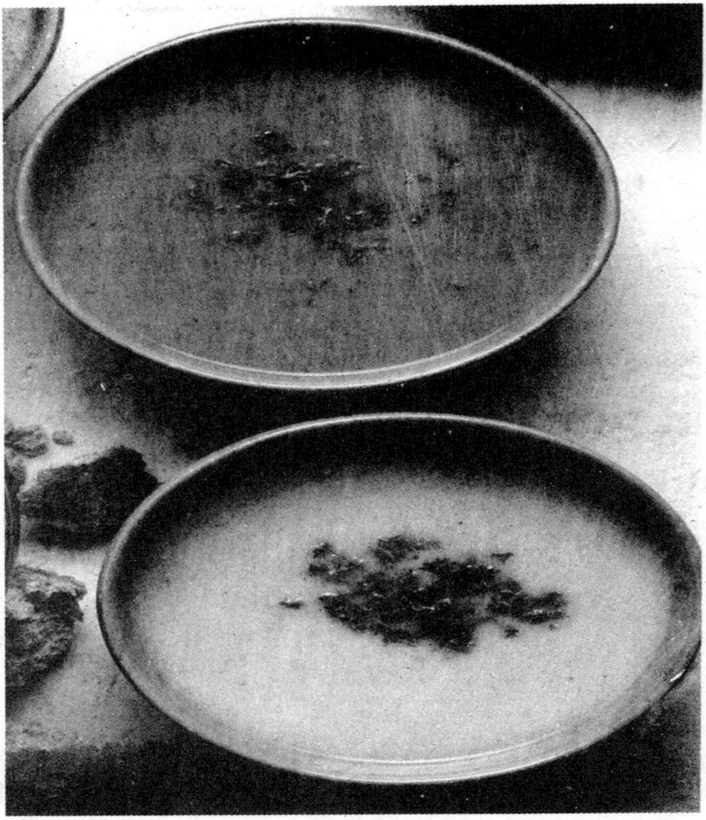

fats, which increase cholesterol (harmful for the heart) in the body.

- Pulses such as lentils, dried peas, soybeans, chick peas and haricot beans provide vegetable protein and are also a source of vitamin B, iron and other minerals.

- Honey is a natural source of sugar and is rich in minerals such as calcium and magnesium.

- Eggs, although high in cholesterol, are very rich in protein and contain vitamins and minerals in good quantities.
- Fish is a particularly important source of protein and contains a wide range of essential vitamins and minerals.

Nutrition Value of Vitamin and Minerals (at a glance)

Vitamin/ Mineral	*Function*	*Daily intake*
Vitamin A	Good for night vision.	5000 IU
Vitamin B_1	Functioning of nervous system, heart, liver.	1.5 mg
Vitamin B_2	Good vision, clear eyes.	2 mg
Vitamin B_3	Breaks down fats, protein. Carbohydrates important for mental health.	15 mg
Vitamin B_5	For functioning of adrenal glands.	-
Vitamin B_6	Aids metabolism, forms antibodies,Red blood cells, nervous system.	2 mg

(Contd.)

(Contd. Table)

Vitamin/ Mineral	*Function*	*Daily intake*
Vitamin C	Maintains essential protein, collagen,Heals wounds, skin care, viral and bacterial infections.	50 mg
Vitamin D	Helps bone building.	400 IU
Vitamin E	Circulation system, ageing process.	20 IU
Vitamin K	Prevent hemorrhaging.	-
Calcium	Builds and maintains bones.	600 mg
Chlorine	Helps cell metabolism.	2-5 g
Chromium	Regulate blood sugar levels.	a trace
Cobalt	Aids Vit. B_{12} , red blood cells.	a trace
Copper	Helps enzymes, red blood cells.	2.5 mg
Fluorine	Strengthen bones, prevent decay.	1 mg
Iodine	Necessary for thyroid hormone.	a trace
Iron	Helps carry oxygen to cells, formation of hemoglobin.	15 mg
Magnesium	Nerve and muscle functioning, Cell metabolism.	300 mg

(Contd.)

(Contd. Table)

Vitamin/ Mineral	*Function*	*Daily intake*
Manganese	Helps blood sugar level, Activates Enzymes, reproductive processes.	A trace
Phosphorus	Growth and repair of cells.	1 g
Potassium	Helps muscle control, water balance.	4 g
Selenium	Anti-oxidant, prevent cancers.	A trace
Sodium	Cellular metabolism, prevent fluid loss.	2.5 g
Sulphur	Helps formation of body tissue, detoxant.	A trace
Zinc	Helps enzymes and proteins, digestion	A trace

Breast Milk

Breast feeding is very important as it helps to build a strong bond between mother and the baby and is also the best form of nourishment for newborn infant. The quantity and the quality of milk produced in breasts is not related to the size of the breast but is dependent on the amount of fluid a feeding mother consume. Breast milk is natural, pure and unadulterated form of nourishment for the child. It provides antibodies to the baby which is why it is superior to the formulae feeds or cow milk. The nutritional quality of breast milk is much higher than that of cow's or buffalo's milk as it contains more lactose (sugar), vitamin A, C and E, fat and iron.

Composition of Food

Product	*Water Contents*	*Protein*	*Fiber*	*Carbohydrate*
Chicken	63 %	20 %	0	0
Fish (Lamb, Mackerel, Pork)	64 %	18 %	0	0
Eggs	74 %	12 %	0	1 %
Bread	36 %	7.8 %	0	50 %
Butter	16 %	0.5 %	0	0.5 %
Cheese	4.2 %	25 %	0	2 %
Milk	87 %	3.5 %	0	4.5 %
Rice	12 %	7 %	1 %	77 %
Peanuts	5 %	16 %	2 %	16 %
Kidney beans	12 %	24 %	4.5 %	55 %
Apple	84 %	0.5 %	2 %	13 %
Grapefruit	88 %	1 %	0.5 %	10 %
Mushrooms	92 %	2 %	5.5 %	0
Cabbage	90 %	3.5 %	1 %	5 %

(Contd.)

(Contd. Table)

Product	*Water Contents*	*Protein*	*Fiber*	*Carbohydrate*
Carrot	89 %	1.5 %	1 %	8 %
Peas	81 %	6 %	1.5 %	11 %
Potatoes	80 %	2 %	0.5 %	17 %
Lettuce	94 %	1.5 %	1 %	3 %
Tomatoes	95 %	0.5 %	1 %	3 %

The Aim of Dieting....... OBESITY ?

Along with poor nutritional habits goes obesity, one of the major problems in society. Hundreds of diets have been worked out to make weight reducing as quick as easy as possible. Most of the dieting programmes are based on reduction of calorie intake and are effective only in the short term. There is no easy answer to weight control. To reduce weight you must reduce your intake of food. Crash diets certainly do this, but they fail to treat nutritional practices as part of the individual's pattern of living. Unless the overweight person can alter his or her eating habits, all efforts will be in vain. Crash dieting can seriously impair an individual's health sometimes irreparably.

Everybody has a natural weight at which they feel comfortable and it varies from individual to individual depending on the height, weight, body type, bones and so on. The aim of dieting should be to find that unnatural weight and stick to it. Excessive dieting to become thin can be extremely harmful. It may lead to serious disorder anorexia nervosa – **a psychiatric illness usually caused by compulsive dieting and resulting in metabolic disorders in women. There are many nutritionally sound diets that an obese person can follow. One of the best is that recommended by a dietician who may be consulted. As a rule, *an overweight person should loose not more than ½ to 1 kg per week* after the first couple of weeks of dieting. Dieting should always go hand in hand with exercise. This not only burns up calories but also tones up the body and helps to redistribute Weight. The most important of all in tackling obesity is the person's mental attitude. A positive approach to the benefits of healthy food and the cultivation of a genuine pleasure in eating it are essential to long-term weight stability.**

Vegetarianism, Vegans and Macrobiotics

The larger group of vegetarians are those who eat eggs, milk and milk products as well as all plant food, but do not eat flesh foods such as meat, fish and poultry. A vegetarian diet can be as healthy as any other – as long as it is well balanced. Eggs, cheese, milk, pulses and nuts are excellent sources of protein. Vegetables and fruit contain all necessary minerals and vitamins. The vegetarians will generally consume less calories than their meat-eating counterpart, so obesity is rarely a problem. The number of fat vegetarians is much lesser that those of non-vegetarians. Overall, the vegetarian diet, with its emphasis on fresh fruit and vegetables is extremely healthy as long as enough protein and fiber are included in it.

The strict vegan will not eat any animal product at all, including milk, eggs or honey. Nutritionally, veganism has certain disadvantages. The diet is deficient in vitamin B_{12}, since this vitamin is found almost entirely in animal products. Lack of this vitamin can cause very serious anemia and degeneration of spinal cord, leading to nervous disorders. The vegan diet also contains little vitamin D, which is important for the development and growth of strong bones, especially in children. On the whole veganism should be accepted only with very careful thought.

Macrobiotics is a philosophically based system, which promotes health through the use of certain nutritional principles. The macrobiotic diet claims to produce 'wholeness' by creating a balance. The macrobiotic diet is centered on cooked grains, cooked vegetables and miso soup. Miso (high in enzymes) is a black paste made from fermented soya beans, sea salt and a grain such as brown rice, believed to be valuable to the digestive system and is a rich source of vitamin B_{12}

The Naturopathic Laws of Hygiene and Health Maintenance

Naturopathy is a holistic therapy and encompasses not only diet – but also various forms of hydrotherapy, massage and exercise. The naturopathic belief is: we have within our own body all resources and means for achieving health, maintaining health and combating disease. The naturopathic laws of hygiene and health maintenance are as following:

- Look for your own health and your body needs.
- Eat moderately and healthily.
- Beware of body, mind and soul – that must be regarded as such in all efforts to achieve total health.
- Avoid use of alcohol and other stimulating drinks.
- Take regular exercise and breath healthily. Encourage yoga for health.
- Avoid stress and resolve stress problems in the environment.
- Ensure proper sleep and rest.
- Select a good diet. Food is an important factor for good health.
- Animal fats contribute to heart disease, blood pressure and breast cancer.

- The naturopathic diet is high in vegetable matter, half of which should be taken raw.
- The vegetables, if possible, should be grown on organically fertilized soil as vegetables grown on artificially fertilized soil and sprayed with chemicals are harmful for health.

Juice Therapy for Slimming

Juice therapy also known as juice fasting is most effective way to restore health and rejuvenate the body. Raw juice therapy is a method of treatment of disease through an exclusive diet of juices of fruit and vegetables. An exclusive diet of raw juices of fruit and vegetables result in much faster and effective recovery from diseases, which cleanse and regenerate the tissues than fasting. Drinking alkali-forming fruit and vegetable juices during fasting increase the healing effect of fasting. All juices should be made fresh immediately before drinking. Raw juices from root vegetables may be combined with those of green leafy vegetables, but not with other juices. A glass of water mixed with lemon juice and 20-30 gm. Honey may be taken first in the morning. Thereafter, the prescribed juice may be taken at three-hourly intervals. The patient should take adequate rest during the raw juice treatment. A proper selection of juice in treating particular ailment is very essential.

18

Pregnancy and Post-natal Body Care

A little everyday care ensures that the natural beauty of your body does not fade away too soon. Here are few basic guidelines to a beauty and body regime a woman can maintain during the period of pregnancy and post-natal.

Posture Problem During Pregnancy

The changes in the menstrual cycle usually occur due to female sex hormones from the regulating center – the pituitary gland influenced by the brain. The pituitary glands stimulate the ovaries to secrete estrogen hormones. The ovaries begin the secretion of progesterone for the preparation of fertilized egg to get settled in the uterus. There is sudden drop in the level of progesterone and estrogen, the inner lining of uterus starts breaking up and escapes out through vagina mixed with blood as menstrual flow. This changing cycle leaves adverse effect on a woman's posture.

Pigmentation of skin is a major problem during periods. What we want is an even toned, translucent, radiant and blemish-free skin and slim-trim body during these days. The melanin in the skin is the culprit. The amount and distribution of this pigment determines skin color and differs. The imbalance in the amount and distribution stay on just the upper layer of the skin or run deep as well. Hyper-pigmentation is usually faced by women during periods, pregnancy and post-natal. The common problems related to pigmentation are Melasma: a brownish discoloration that usually starts after pregnancy, usually seen on the face (cheeks, forehead and nose) and other parts of the body, but tends to persist till the delivery of infant and lactating period. There are several treatments available, to cope with pigmentation and your posture, you can select one according to the recommendation of your doctor.

Beauty Tips for Pregnant

Pregnancy can change your appearance due to rapid hormonal changes, which cause dry, flaky skin or a blotchy acne-prone complexion. Body undergoes many changes including severe fatness during pregnancy. Skin is the first thing to bear the burn of it. Some of the common problems include very dry, itchy skin, melasma, acne and stretch marks. Do not despair, these can be treated during and after pregnancy. Usually, from the second trimester of pregnancy, a pregnant woman might suddenly find herself with very dry, taut skin that is sand papery to the touch, especially around the stomach, breasts, hands and legs. Do not be alarmed, generally the condition vanishes after delivery. But till then be sure to keep skin extra moisturized with a creamy body lotion. Almond oil or cocoa butter based creams tend to work wonders in soothing the skin during this period when applied after bath.

Stretch, Marks on Face and Body

For most women the skin tends to clear up during pregnancy due to extra blood flow in the system. Few women give rise to acne and pimples. Stretch marks are undoubtedly the biggest

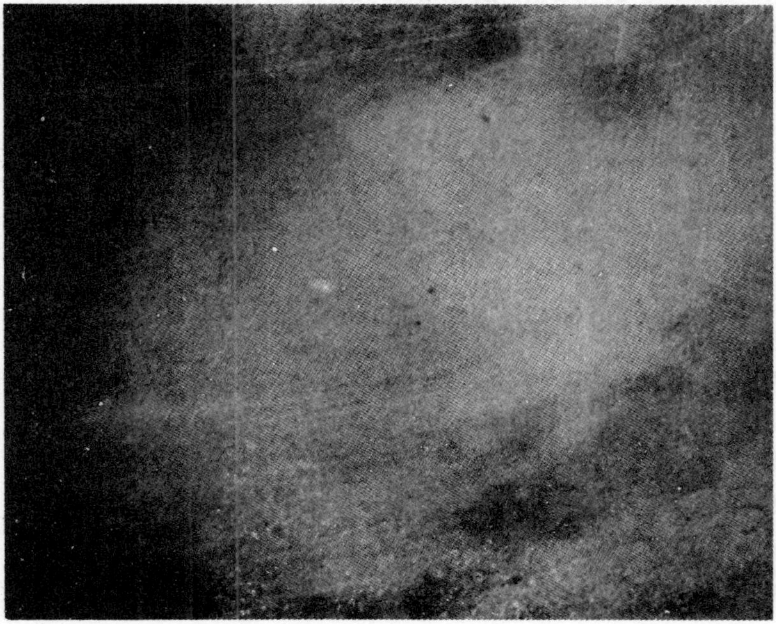

problem that almost all pregnant women worry about. This happens when the skin loses its elasticity due to the stretching of the upper and lower layers of the skin. They generally appear as red marks, which form white strip-like marks across stomach. With timely treatment and massage with vitamin E oil accompanied by a balanced diet, the stretch marks may lighten.

The First Three Months

Pregnancy can also be a time of difficulty for a mother-to-be. There are additional physical strains to cope with along with confusing and conflicting advice from friends and relatives. In the midst of such pressures, a pregnant woman often has no room for her beauty and body care. But it is very important for an expectant woman to spend some of her times thinking about herself. If the expectant mother is relaxed and healthy, then her baby stands a good chance of being healthy too. The 40 weeks of pregnancy have several beauty and body problems as well as some beauty bonuses. Nature may prove very good for some mothers-to-be. They may find that pregnancy produces unexpected benefits like clear skin, glowing cheeks, glossy hair and attractive body. An expectant mother may become beautiful, if she starts taking extra beauty care from the very beginning.

During the first trimester of pregnancy, there is great hormonal activity in the body. The figure becomes plump and lumpy. The joy of realizing that you are going to be a mother may be clouded by doubts and disappointment over the way you look disfigured. Start by thinking positive about your beauty care and a daily beauty routine. Spots appearing on the face, chest or back should not worry you as the increased hormonal activity in your body is causing this temporary upset. Never squeeze any spot anywhere on your body to get rid of it, which may leave a permanent scar. When you are pregnant, pay special attention to lubricate the skin on your stomach, buttocks and breasts. Apply plenty of skin conditioning cream after your bath and rub in baby oil or olive oil every night. Stretch marks are very difficult remove after the birth of baby. Lubrication of the skin at this time can prevent spots and wrinkles and pay handsome dividend later on. Keep lubricating throughout the nine months of pregnancy period.

You need more attention on your diet in this period. You need more nutrients, not more calories. Cut out fried, sweet and fatty foods. If you are non-vegetarian, fish provides Vitamin D, which you need at this stage. Drink a glass of milk a day, it fulfils the need of Calcium. Take smaller meals more frequently during the day. Avoid really strenuous exercise during the crucial first three months. Go to the bed early. The most radiant mother-to-be of all is the rested one.

The Second Trimester

Beauty and body care taken early in pregnancy now begins to pay dividends. Hair and skin conditions improve at this stage. Continue with daily stomach, bottom and breast lubrication and pay special attention to skin freshness. Underarm depilation and deodorizing are essential. Night cramps are often a problem at this stage. Keep strict watch on your diet and weight gain. Total weight gain during pregnancy should be about 12 kg. Remember, toxaemia (blood poisoning) and high blood pressure are dangers for overweight mothers-to-be, and so are varicose veins. Keep walking with your doctor's advice. Walk slowly. It is important to keep up light exercise as per your doctor's approval. Going to bed early during this period is a good habit to enhance grooming of your body. The most comfortable position in bed is lying on your side with one leg slightly in front of the other, one hand under the pillow, and the other by your side. That way the weight is evenly distributed.

The Final Months

This is the time for the final preparations to welcome the baby. Take good care of yourself too, you will need a lot of energy in the coming months to bring up baby as well as to retain your beauty and posture. Dryness and blotchiness are sometimes problems at the end of pregnancy period. Take care to nourish your skin rightly.

Give your body plenty of skin cream in the last two months. If you intend to breastfeed your baby, keep your nipples soft with a special cream to help prevent cracking and massage breasts to avoid over-development and fat.

Increase milk and high protein food in your diet. Keep your iron intake high, too. Drink fresh orange juice instead of tea or coffee. A high Vitamin C intake helps protect you against infections. When labor begins, have a good meal. A good sleep is necessary during the final month.

Post-natal Care of Your Beauty and Body

Having a baby takes a great deal of energy. Even though you have been following a good anti-natal beauty programme you are bound to feel tired and exhausted for first few months after the birth of child. Make sure that your diet is rich in nutrients such as plenty of vitamin C, protein and minerals. Keep up the iron supplement you took before baby was born. Take care of your body and have regular exercise, otherwise you will loose shape of your body.

The Pelvis

Before becoming pregnant for the first time many women are surprisingly unaware of the internal workings of their own bodies. However, once the pregnancy is confirmed, the pelvis and its associated muscles and organs become the center of interest and it is important to understand the role of the pelvis in pregnancy and childbirth. The bones of the pelvis form the strong frame that acts like a cradle, surrounding, supporting and protecting the womb.

The pelvic floor is the essential sling of muscle that helps to hold the pelvic organs in place. Several layers of, the pelvic muscles are slung under the pelvis in two intersecting circles, which look like a figure 'Eight (8)'. The larger, top ring of the muscle controls the outlets of the urethral and vaginal sphincters. Below is the smaller circle of muscle, which contains the stronger anal or rectal, sphincter. The muscles overlap and so they are thicker at the perineum, the area between the anus and vagina.

Pelvic floor exercises are important throughout your life. Sensitivity in this area increases your love making enjoyment. If the muscles become slack you will find that you lack enjoy during sexual intercourse as much and may have difficulty reaching orgasm. Your male partner will also find love making less enjoyable. Remember, a weak pelvic floor can lead to incontinence and even prolapse, and sagging of the walls of the vagina.

Pelvis Exercises

The following movements will help you prepare the pelvic area for childbirth. Practice these movements daily in rhythmic slow motion, repeating each for five to six times. These simple exercises will help provide you the best position for yourself and your baby during labor.

1. *Pelvic tilt (Standing Position)*: The pelvic tilt is an essential movement for maintaining good posture during pregnancy and after the birth. Tilt your pelvis by lifting the pubic bone up in front, the abdominal and buttock muscles are most effectively able to support the trunk and minimize strain on your lower back. To do this exercise, stand with your feet little way from the wall, hip width apart, bend knees slightly and rest your back, shoulders and head against the wall. Breathe in. As you breathe out, press your lower back firmly against the wall, pulling in your abdomen and lifting your pubic bone, so your buttocks tighten and leave the wall. Keep shoulders pressed against the wall and move the pelvis only.

2. *Pelvic tilt (Second Posture)*: Kneel with your knees in line with your hips and hands in line with your shoulders. Keep your back flat. Now pull in your abdominal muscles, tighten your buttocks and do a pelvic tilt, so your back humps up. Do not rock your pubic bone back in this position or when lean forwards, that might strain your back.

3. *Dancing Exercise*: Dancing is an excellent exercise. Rocking and circling the pelvis are basic movements in all rhythmic dance. You may dance to music either standing or kneeling or on all fours circling the pelvis. The regular practice of this exercise helps comfort during labor.

Spine

The spine is the supporting structure of the body connecting your head, ribs, pelvis and limbs. Between each movable joint of the spine is a soft jelly-like disc that allows freedom of the movement. If you allow your spine to sag, these soft discs may become squashed causing stiffness and pain. Muscles of the back, too, help you to keep the spine lengthen. If your back is stiff and inflexible, loosen it up with the exercises as detailed in this chapter. Gently twisting your back is relaxing and invigorating and helps to prevent you straining. Stretch out your back with pelvic tilt before you start exercising. Spinal Exercises are the following:

1. Stretch your spine sitting, standing or lying down. Practice the movement sitting against a wall. Pull your shoulder blades together and down. Then press your back against the wall, giving a pelvic tilt. Get into the habit of practicing this movement whenever you settle into a chair or car seat.

2. Sit against the wall pressing your back. Now stretch your arms above your head at the same time, flattening them as far back as you can against the wall. Keep your shoulders down.

3. Kneel with your knees hip-width apart. Slowly twist to the right. Hold for a moment; then repeat to the left. Prevent twisting your hips and thighs.

4. Sit cross-legged. Press against your knee to help you twist farther.

5. Stand straight, both knees facing forward. Swing your arms for extra momentum and twist from side to side standing.

Strengthen Your Back

Try to straighten your back, as the straightening motion strengthens the back muscles. 'Tailor sitting' strengthens the muscles of back as described below:

Tailor sitting position is useful in preparation for labor as it loosens the groin and hips, and stretches the muscles of the inner thighs. It also stimulates the circulation in the lower half of the body. Practicing this will help you to hold a variety of positions in labor and will let your legs flop wide apart during the delivery of child. The following is the procedure for Tailor sitting:

1. Sit on the floor with the soles of your feet together.
2. Hold your ankles.
3. Bring your pelvis and feet as close together as you can by walking forward on your hips.
4. Keep your back straight.
5. In case you feel uncomfortable in practicing this posture, place a couple of cushions under each of your thighs for support.

Lying down position: You may try this posture in lying down position. Practice Tailor sit posture and lean backward slowly till your back touches the floor. You can seek the help of your partner while leaning backward, and coming to initial Tailor sitting position after few seconds.

Exercises to Strengthen Your Back

1. Sit against a wall to feel the length of your spine. Lift knees upward so that the soles of both feet press each other. This is also a good way to check whether your back is really straight.

2. Sit straight without giving support of wall. Prop yourself up with your arms on the floor to help you lift. Make a loose fist with each hand and press the fist into the floor behind you as you lift your ribs away from the hips and straighten your back. Make sure that shoulders do not move up.

Sitting, Leg Apart for Slimming Lower Body

This exercise stretches the groin, inside thighs, back of the legs and strengthens the quadriceps – the muscles at the front of the thighs. This exercise is particularly important in pregnancy when the extra weight can put undue strain on the knees. The exercise strengthens the muscles and also helps you to cope with the weight

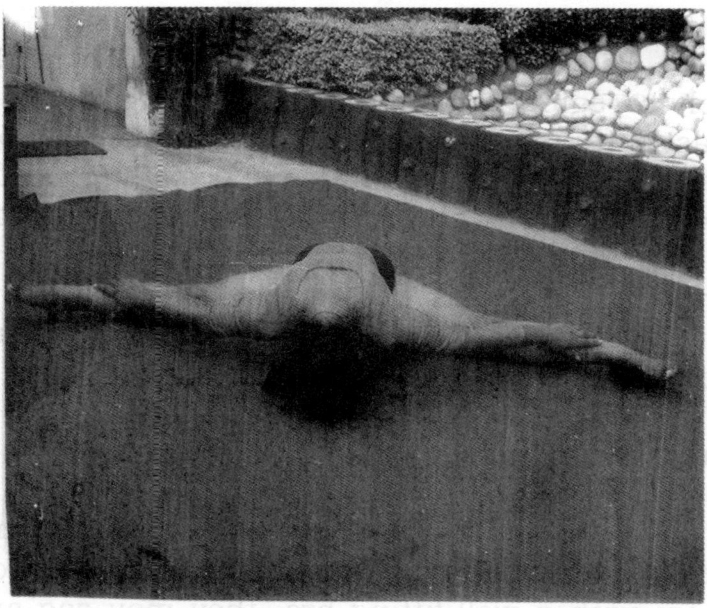

of the baby. To practice this exercise, following movements are applied:

1. Sit straight, lifting your back.
2. Wide your legs as much as you can sideways, one leg at a time.

3. Tighten the muscles of your legs and keep toes pointing upwards.
4. Now hook big toes with your index and middle fingers. If hands doesn't touch the feet, take them up to the point you do comfortably.
5. Bend forward and rest your forehead or chin on the floor. If it is uncomfortable, do not practice this exercise. Do not bend your knees.

This exercise improves circulation in the pelvic region and makes hamstring muscles elastic. It makes delivery easier and relieves labor pains. The exercises is also especially good for women other than pregnant for curing all menstruation disorder, strengthen genital organs and increases sex power. The exercise keeps joints, muscles, organs and nerves strong and healthy besides slimming the body.

Breasts

Your breasts are likely to become larger and heavier during pregnancy, and unless you support them with a well-fitting bra, they may sag and lose their shape. So even if you don't normally wear a bra, you should do so while your breasts are heavy. There are no muscles in the breasts themselves, but you can help to maintain their shape by exercising the muscle underneath. Here are few exercises/ massage movements for breast beauty:

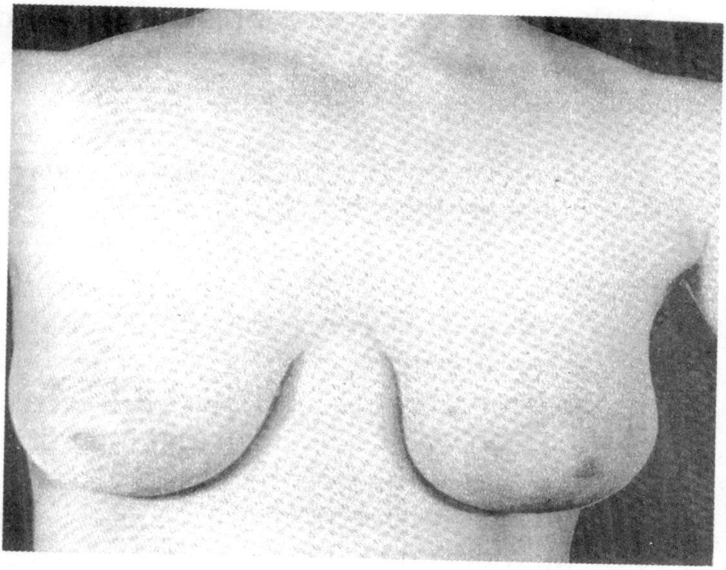

1. Make a loose fist with one hand and clasp the other round it. Hold your hands level

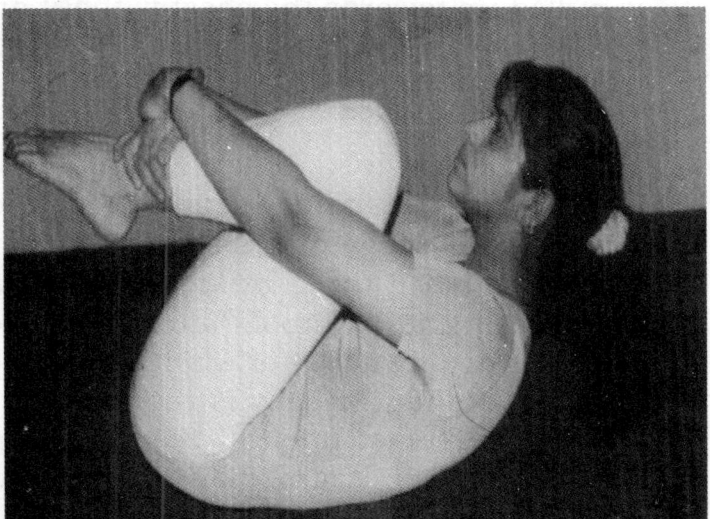

with your breasts and press your hands together tightly for few moments. Repeat the sequence several times.

2. Lie on your back. Pull knees up towards the chest without any pull on ankles. Stay in this position for 6-8 seconds, release the knees on the floor and repeat for three to four times. This exercise strengthens the muscles of the upper part of the body including breasts, relieves lines and wrinkles on waist, abdomen and intestines. Practice of this exercise tones up the muscles of abdomen and intestine, cures constipation and gastric trouble, corrects malfunctioning of stomach, helps uterus come to original position during childbirth. This exercise can also be done in standing position during post-natal, when the knee is pulled up towards the chest without any pull on ankles by one leg at a time. Stay in this position for 6-8 seconds.

3. Massage helps to re-shape your breasts which start expanding during pregnancy and become saggy and shapeless during post-natal when the baby feeds. A regular massage in the bathroom after shower or bath during pregnancy or when the mother is breastfeeding the baby is very helpful to strengthen breast muscle. Start massage making slow, gentle strokes with both hands over the bulge.

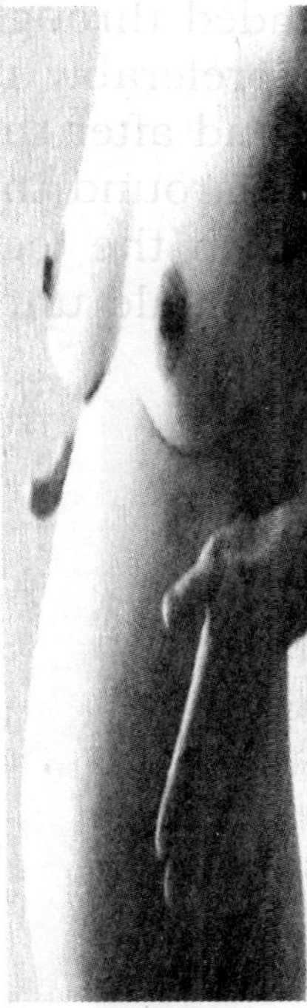

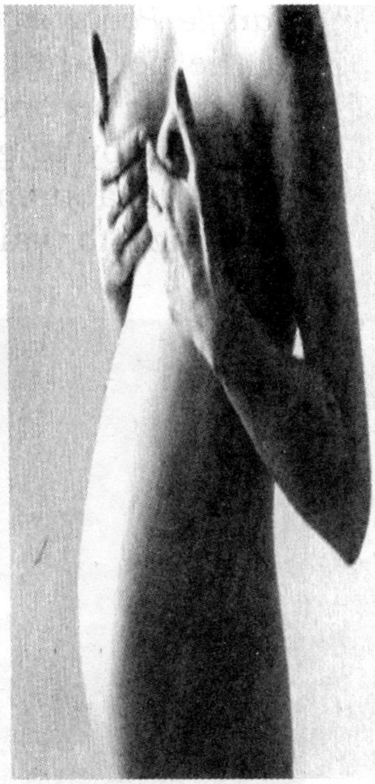

Abdomen

Strong abdominal muscles help you carry the baby more easily without straining your back. They are also helpful during the birth, when the baby is being pushed out; better the condition of your abdomen muscles the easier it is to restore them afterward. The following exercises/ massage movements help strengthening the abdominal muscles:

1. The most important exercise for the abdomen muscles is simply to pull in your abdomen as you breathe out, as often as you can.

2. *Triangle Posture*: is recommended through out the period of pregnancy (preferably in the first or second trimester) and after the birth of baby to get rid of flab around the waist and abdomen. Stand with the legs apart. Rotate waist, begin to exhale until

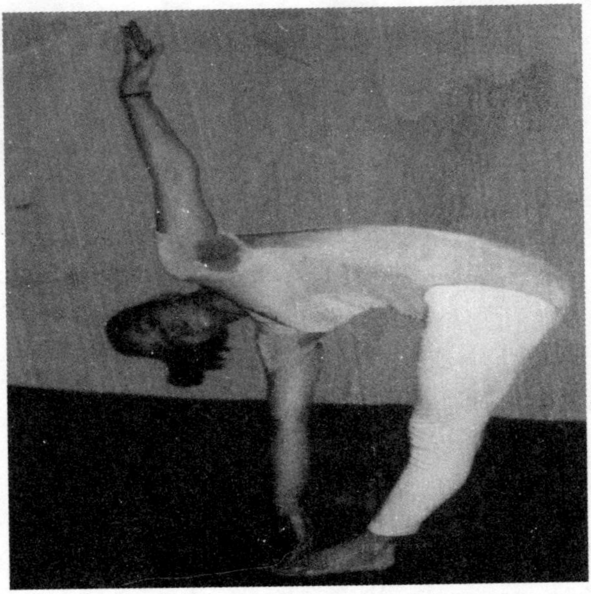

the fingers of the right hand touch the ground. Hold for some time, stand up and perform the same movement to the other hand. This posture makes the entire body strong and elastic, and also toning the muscles in the back, hips and legs.

3. *Sun Exercise*: Stand straight with arms on sides. Raise both arms upward, stretched. Inhale slowly, bend downward and touch

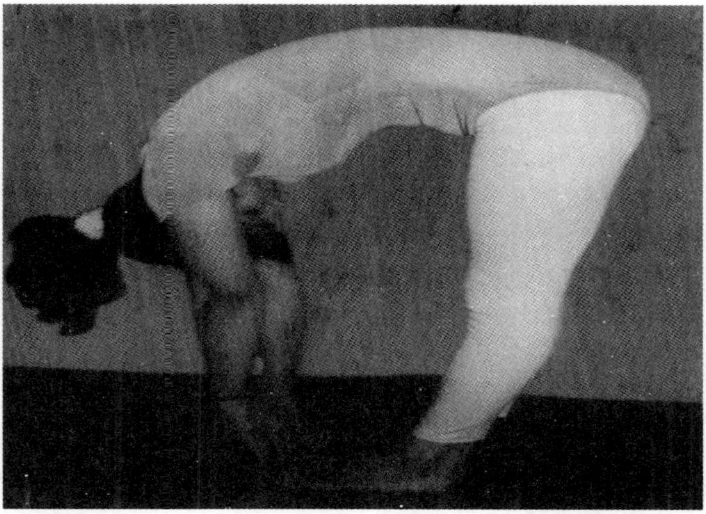

the floor with both hands. This posture tones up the muscles of abdomen, waist, hips and relieve extra fat from these areas. The exercise is especially beneficial after the birth of baby.

4. *Curl ups Exercises*: These movements are beneficial throughout pregnancy, except perhaps during the last few weeks. Continue curl ups movements as long as they are not uncomfortable. Just remember not to strain, if you feel pressure on the pelvic floor, the exercise is too strenuous.

   To practice this exercise, lie on your back with your legs bent, feet hip-width apart, your hands on your thighs. Breathe in. As you breathe out raise your head and shoulders, dropping your chin and reaching

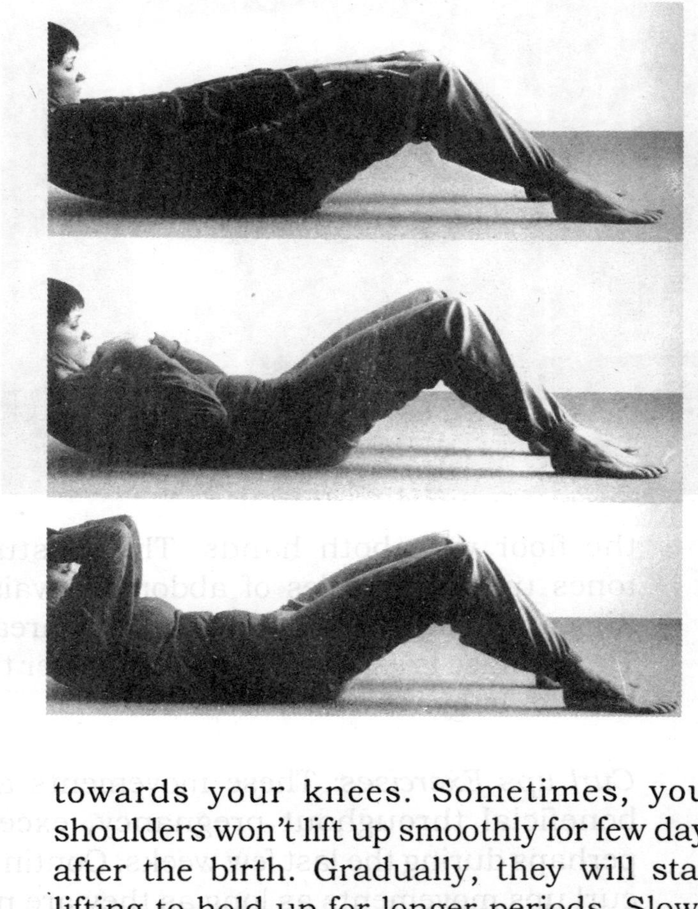

towards your knees. Sometimes, your shoulders won't lift up smoothly for few days after the birth. Gradually, they will start lifting to hold up for longer periods. Slowly progress to resting your hands on chest and clasping hands behind the head.

5. *Leg rolls movement*: This exercise is practiced in the same way as above lying on the back with legs bent, knees together. Lower the knees on the floor and sideways giving movements to the abdomen and legs slowly.

6. *Sides bends*: In this movement, lie on your back, legs straight and together with your arms at your sides and palms flat on the thighs. Lift your head and bend to the right. Rest. Lift head and return to the center. Rest. Lift head and bend to the left and return to the center after having rest. Repeat the whole process three to four times.

7. *Kneel on movement*: Kneel on all fours, your knees in line with your hips and your hands in line with your shoulders. This exercise

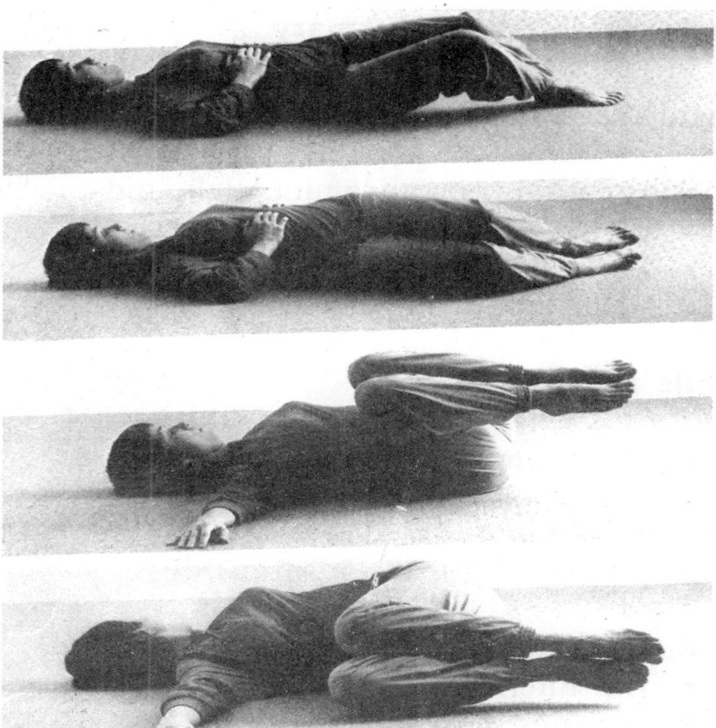

comprises of stretched leg movements in all directions and walking on all fours. This is a beneficial postnatal exercise.

Abdominal massage is very essential to avoid lines and wrinkles during the third trimester of pregnancy Start massage from lower abdomen making slow, gentle, circular strokes with both hands over the bulge. This is particularly comforting towards the end of pregnancy. Start again at the sides, using the same strokes, continue up to under the breast fold.

Postnatal Exercise Summary

Basic Essentials

- Breathing and abdominal tightening, Pelvic tilt
- Pelvic floor exercise
- Relaxation, lying face down

While in Bed

- Stretching movements
- Foot pedaling and circling

During End of First Week After Delivery

- Leg sliding exercises
- Hip hitching
- Leg rolls movements

During Second Week After the Delivery

- Curl down movements
- Curl ups movements
- Leg rolls movements
- Diagonal curl ups movements
- Side bends exercises

Buttocks

The buttocks play an essential part in supporting the trunk and the growing weight of the baby as together with the abdominal muscles, they control the tilt of your pelvis. As the abdominal muscles become stretched because of the growing bulge in front, you have to depend more on buttocks to keep correct posture and prevent low back pain. Strong buttocks may also help to prevent sciatica. If they are flabby and collect a lot of fat, or if they protrude at the sides of your thighs, you can take it that they need strengthening of muscles. The simplest exercise is to squeeze your buttocks together slowly for some time.

Here is another a bit tough exercise for the buttocks:

Lie on your back with your legs bent, feet hip-width apart. Do a pelvic tilt and continue pushing your hips up until your back is in straight line from shoulders to knees. Hold the position for few moments, squeezing your buttocks tightly together. Hold for few seconds, and lower the hips. Repeat three times, twice a day. You can also do this exercise when you are resting on the floor with your legs on a low sofa or bed, keeping the legs straight.

Legs and Feet

Unless your legs and feet are strong, the extra weight you are carrying make them tired resulting cramps and varicose veins. Strong muscles help to prevent cramps, varicose veins and will make your legs feel less sluggish. Exercises stimulate the blood flow in the nerves, is particularly helpful. Here is an exercise to stimulate the nerves of legs:

Stand straight with your feet together. Hold wall or a table for balance. Rise up on the balls of your feet. Do a pelvic tilt. Clench your buttocks tightly together. Do several small bends until you are tired. Stand up straight again.

Cramps

These can be very painful and annoying if they wake you up in the middle of the night. There is no proven remedy, but you might try a calcium and vitamin D supplement or extra milk. If the cramps are in the feet, bend it upward. When the cramps subside, do some ankle circles to stimulate the circulation.

Varicose Veins

The extra progesterone in your body relaxes the muscles in the walls of your veins, increasing the risk of varicose veins developing. These can appear on the legs or in the vulva (the opening of vagina) or in the anal passage, where they are called hemorrhoids. Take care to avoid constipation in such case. If hemorrhoids is neglected,it can be very painful.

Aching Legs

Try to rest with your feet up. Do some leg exercise as well. Swimming and walking are both excellent exercises. Gentle massage on the legs may help and relieve pain.

Massage

Touching, stroking and holding are the most direct ways of communicating with those you love. During the last stage of pregnancy you need a massage by your partner with talcum powder, moisturizer or massage oil on bare skin. Sit on the chair leaning forward on to a cushion. Leaning forward takes the weight of infant in womb, off the lower back. To start massage, ask your partner to rest hands on your shoulder and upper back squeezing with thumbs, sliding hands downwards on either side of spine. Stroke with slowly and firmly up the length of the spine, ending at the base of the skull.

Index